Doping and Public Health

Doping – the use of performance-enhancing substances and methods – has long been a high-profile issue in sport but in recent years it has also become an issue in wider society. This important new book examines doping as a public health issue, drawing on a multi-disciplinary set of perspectives to explore the prevalence, significance and consequences of doping in wider society. It introduces the epidemiology of doping, examines the historical context, and explores the social, behavioral, legal, ethical and political aspects of doping. The book also discusses possible interventions for addressing the problem on organizational and societal levels.

Doping and Public Health incorporates the latest research to provide a comprehensive guide to the key aspects of doping as a social phenomenon. Divided into six parts, this collection of studies offers detailed insight into:

- ideals of health and fitness in today's society
- reasons behind the use of doping
- medical and social consequences of doping
- the importance of a doping-free society
- challenges to the detection and prevention of doping
- the global anti-doping movement.

This book is a valuable resource for sport students, instructors and sport professionals, and will also be of interest to educators and policy-makers working in the areas of health, criminology, sociology and law.

Nader Ahmadi has a PhD in sociology and is Associate Professor and Vice President of the University of Gävle, Sweden. His research has mainly focused on areas such as welfare and social policy, international social work, identity and youth problems, coping strategies among cancer patients, socio-cultural perceptions of the self and gender roles, etc. He has been consultant for the World Bank, UNICEF and the European Commission in many countries such as Russia, Croatia, Vietnam, Azerbaijan, Tajikistan, FYR of Macedonia, Kosovo and Bosnia and Herzegovina. He has also been leader of a nationwide research project on the health problems among the asylum-seeking children in Sweden commissioned by the Swedish government. Ahmadi has been guest lecturer in India, China and Russia.

Arne Ljungqvist – medical professor, high jumper and sports manager – has devoted his life to the service of medicine and sports. He managed to become the Swedish champion in high jump as well as participate in the Helsinki 1952 Olympics. Among other roles he has been Chairman of the Department of Pathology and Cytology, Karolinska Hospital; Pro Rector at the Karolinska Institute, Sweden; President of Swedish Cancer Society; Chairman of the International Olympic Committee's (IOC) Medical Commission; founder and Vice Chairman of the World Anti-Doping Agency (WADA); Chairman of the WADA Health, Medical and Research Committee. In 2014 he received an honorary doctorate from the Faculty of Health and Occupational Studies at the University of Gävle, Sweden.

Göran Svedsäter has a Specialization degree in Psychology and Science of Education and is currently Lecturer at the University of Gävle, Sweden. He has been Lecturer and Leader of Research and Development at the Faculty of Education and Health Care Education, Oslo College, and Lecturer at the Faculty of Health Care Education, College of Trondheim. He has also been consultant for International Doping Tests & Management (testing activities, recruiting, education and training of international sampling officers). He also has experience as doping control officer for the Norwegian Confederation of Sport and as an international doping control officer for several international federations.

Doping and Public Health

Edited by Nader Ahmadi,
Arne Ljungqvist and Göran Svedsäter

Routledge
Taylor & Francis Group
LONDON AND NEW YORK

First published 2016 by Routledge

2 Park Square, Milton Park, Abingdon, Oxfordshire OX14 4RN
711 Third Avenue, New York, NY 10017

Routledge is an imprint of the Taylor & Francis Group, an informa business

First issued in paperback 2017

British Library Cataloguing-in-Publication Data
A catalogue record for this book is available from the British Library

Library of Congress Cataloging in Publication Data
A catalog record for this book has been requested

ISBN: 978-1-138-91855-9 (hbk)
ISBN: 978-1-138-57430-4 (pbk)

Typeset in Times New Roman
by Wearset Ltd, Boldon, Tyne and Wear

Contents

Illustrations

Figures

Tables

Contributors

Nader Ahmadi has a PhD in sociology and is Associate Professor and Vice president of the University of Gävle, Sweden. His research has mainly focused on areas such as welfare and social policy, international social work, identity and youth problems, coping strategies among cancer patients, socio-cultural perceptions of the self and gender roles, etc. He has been consultant for the World Bank, UNICEF and the European Commission in many countries such as Russia, Croatia, Vietnam, Azerbaijan, Tajikistan, FYR of Macedonia, Kosovo and Bosnia and Herzegovina. He has also been leader of a nationwide research project on the health problems among asylum-seeking children in Sweden commissioned by the Swedish government. Ahmadi has been guest lecturer in India, China and Russia.

Timothy Armstrong is a Coordinator at the Department of Prevention of Non-Communicable Diseases at the World Health Organization (WHO) in Geneva. He has managed the Global Strategy on Diet and Physical Activity within the WHO and is responsible for the WHO Commission on Ending Childhood Obesity.

Nicolas Clark is a Medical Officer with the Management of Substance Abuse Team at the World Health Organization in Geneva and has published extensively on the topic of substance abuse.

Clément de Maillard is a PhD candidate at the Ecole de Sciences Criminelles, Université de Lausanne, Switzerland, and project manager for INTERPOL Anti-doping Project.

Theodore Friedmann is MD and Professor of Pediatrics at the University of California, San Diego, La Jolla. He is also Muriel Jeanette Whitehill Chair in Biomedical Ethics at UCSD. Friedmann has won many awards, among them the University of California Chancellor's Association Award for Excellence in Research. He has been Consultant on Gene Therapy to the Swedish Royal Academy, Chairman, Scientific Advisory Board, L/N Syndrome Children's Res. Foundation, Elected Fellow at the American Association for the Advancement of Science, and Member of the IOC, WADA, Committee of Medicine, Health and Research and the US Anti-Doping Agency.

Hans Geyer is a managing director at the Centre for Preventive Doping Research, German Sport University in Cologne. He is also the deputy head of the WADA-accredited doping control laboratory in Cologne, Germany. Since 1983 he has worked in the field of doping research, especially in the development of methods for the detection of anabolic steroids and in the analysis of nutritional supplements for doping substances.

David Hoff is Senior Lecturer in Social Work at the School of Social Work, Lund University, Sweden, and is also affiliated with the University of Gävle. Hoff has a PhD in Sociology of Law. His main research interests include different perspectives on doping in sport as well as outside the sporting context (e.g. as a social issue). The focus of his research is on individual and social driving forces for doping in relation to processes and trends in society. Hoff has also written about the system of governance in relation to doping in sport from a sociology of law perspective.

Mathieu Holz is a Master of Criminal Law and has been Captain of the French Gendarmerie Nationale and a Criminal Intelligence Officer at the General Secretariat of INTERPOL. Holz has also been in charge of doping matters in a cooperation between the World Anti-Doping Agency (WADA) and INTERPOL.

David Howman commenced work for WADA as Chief Operating Officer/ Special Counsel in March 2003, and has been Director General for WADA since 2003.

Arne Ljungqvist, medical professor, high jumper and sports manager, has devoted his life to the service of medicine and sports. He managed to become the Swedish champion in high jump as well as participate in the Helsinki 1952 Olympics. Among other roles he has been Chairman Department of Pathology and Cytology, Karolinska Hospital; Pro Rector at the Karolinska Institute, Sweden; President of Swedish Cancer Society; Chairman of the International Olympic Committee's (IOC) Medical Commission; founder and Vice Chairman of the World Anti-Doping Agency (WADA); Chairman of the WADA Health, Medical and Research Committee. In 2014 he received an honorary doctorate from the Faculty of Health and Occupational Studies at the University of Gävle, Sweden.

Sigmund Loland is a professor of Sport Philosophy and Ethics at the Norwegian School of Sport Sciences (NSSS). He is widely published in the area of doping and performance-enhancing technologies. Loland is a former Rector of NSSS, a former President of the European College of Sport Science, and a member of WADA's Ethical Issues Review Board.

Michael J. McNamee is Professor of Applied Ethics, Department of Philosophy, History and Law, School of Health Science, Swansea University. He has pioneered the Philosophy of Sport and Sports Ethics as a credible teaching and research field in the UK. He is currently Vice Chair of the European

Association of the Philosophy of Sport. He has served on the Executive Committees of the Philosophy of Education Society of Great Britain, the European College of Sport Science and the International Council for Sport Science and Physical Education. His research interests include ethical issues regarding doping and other human enhancement technologies, research ethics and sports medicine ethics. He is co-editor of Routledge's Ethics and Sport series. He has lectured and published widely on the subject and has developed curricula in the area for a number of UK higher education institutions. Mike McNamee is editor of the journal *Sport, Ethics and Philosophy.*

Thomas H. Murray is President Emeritus of The Hastings Center and formerly Director of the Center for Biomedical Ethics at the School of Medicine at Case Western Reserve University, USA, where he was also the Susan E. Watson Professor of Bioethics. He serves on many editorial boards and has been president of the Society for Health and Human Values and of the American Society for Bioethics and Humanities. He served as the Chair of the Ethical Issues Review Panel for the World Anti-Doping Agency and as International Expert Advisor to Singapore's Bioethics Advisory Committee. Murray is the author of more than 250 publications. In 2004 he received an honorary doctorate from the medical faculty of Uppsala University.

Letizia Paoli is Full Professor of Criminology at the University of Leuven Faculty of Law, Belgium. She was a senior research fellow at the Max Planck Institute for Foreign and International Criminal Law in Freiburg, Germany. She has also been visiting scholar or professor at the Universities of Giessen, Tübingen, Paris I (Sorbonne) and Rotterdam. Since the 1990s she has published extensively on the Italian mafia, organized crime, illegal drugs and related control policies. Since 2010 her research agenda has also included the supply of doping products and anti-doping policy. Between 2010 and 2016 Prof. Paoli chaired a commission of inquiry set up by the University of Freiburg to investigate alleged doping practices at the Freiburg University Sports Medicine Department, which used to train most of West German athletes.

Göran Svedsäter has a Specialization degree in Psychology and Science of Education and is currently Lecturer at the University of Gävle, Sweden. He has been Lecturer and Leader of Research and Development at the Faculty of Education and Health Care Education, Oslo College, and Lecturer at the Faculty of Health Care Education, College of Trondheim. He has also been consultant for International Doping Tests & Management (testing activities, recruiting, education and training of international sampling officers). He also has experience as doping control officer for the Norwegian Confederation of Sport and as an international doping control officer for several international federations.

Elena Titova joined INTERPOL in 2013. She is now specifically dedicated to the criminal intelligence initiative on performance-enhancing drugs trafficking and a member of the INTERPOL Anti-doping Project.

Ivan Waddington is Professor at the University of Chester, UK, and a visiting professor at the Norwegian School of Sport Sciences, Oslo. He is an internationally recognized expert on drugs in sport. He has written more than 90 scholarly papers, including more than 20 on the subject of drugs in sport. His work has been translated into German, French, Italian, Portuguese and Flemish.

Introduction

Doping and public health

Nader Ahmadi, Arne Ljungqvist and Göran Svedsäter

The concept of "doping" is usually associated with sport, particularly elite sport. In fact, doping means the use of substances or methods that are banned in sport by the World Anti-Doping Agency (WADA) because of their potentially performance-enhancing effects. Their use is, therefore, considered to be against the fair play spirit of sport and can also include significant health risks for the user.

However, the use of many doping substances is no longer limited to the world of sport. Doping substances such as anabolic androgenic steroids (AAS) are nowadays used also by people who are not competitive athletes but who want to make use of the effects of AAS in making their bodies more muscular, stronger and impressive in conformity with the current masculine body ideal.

The use of AAS and similar substances appears to be growing and has been found in a range of countries previously not researched. At least, recent data obtained from customs seizures, court cases and some surveys suggest that the extent of AAS use outside sport has been underestimated, some reasons probably being an underground circulation of such drugs in the gym and fitness culture and the easy availability of them on the internet.

One particular concern is the increasing use of nutritional supplements by growing segments of society. A significant percentage of these products have been shown to contain prohibited substances such as steroids that are not listed on the label. This shows that the nutritional supplement industry needs to be more strictly regulated. Until that happens, supplements of dubious value, content and quality will continue to be easily available around the world.

What, then, are the possible reasons that active and health-conscious individuals are willing to take the risk to use preparations such as AAS? A review of the research shows that the most important motive behind the use of AAS outside the elite sports environment, i.e., in a fitness context, is to improve physical appearance. Although most users are boys and young and middle-aged men, also women of various ages use doping substances. Different types of slimming pills are popular among women (including hormone preparations), but possibly even more interesting are the new female fitness and appearance ideals that are connected to muscles and strength. The body has become increasingly important for saying something about who we are. The hunt for the perfect appearance creates a situation where denial instead of acceptance of one's own body influences the individual's self-image.

Doping and public health

In Stockholm in September 2012, an international Symposium entitled "Doping as a public health issue," took place. The Symposium was organized by the Professor Arne Ljungqvist Anti-Doping Foundation and revealed that there is reason to believe that the use of doping substances, in particular AAS, has become a significant public health issue. At the Symposium, several of the world's key stakeholders, including INTERPOL, IOC, UNESCO, WADA and WHO discussed how a new strategy could be developed, coordinated, implemented and monitored for preventing and combating the use of doping substances in sport as well as in the broader society. Some topics that were a part of the contributions and discussions during the seminar are more thoroughly described in this book.

Surveys of doping outside sport are relatively limited in number and there is a need for social science research which can contribute to a better understanding of why and to what extent individuals who are not competitive athletes use doping. From a public health as well as a sports perspective, information, education, research and appropriate legislation and policies are essential components for effective anti-doping actions.

This book will hopefully be a useful resource for anyone who wishes to have a deeper insight into the problem of doping in sport and the larger issue of the use of doping substances in the broader community. In particular, the book is intended for university and college-level students in fields like sports sciences, nursing, sociology, psychology, health promotion, etc., and people who are directly or indirectly involved in the work against the use of doping in sport and society.

The book content

The book is structured around different themes dividing the chapters into those identifying the problem; those presenting explanations; and those making policy recommendations.

Arne Ljungqvist gives a historical account of how the anti-doping work in sport got started in the 1960s, experienced great difficulties during the Cold War era and later received increased support from sport and society which led to the creation of WADA in 1999. He also explains how the use of doping developed from a concern for sport to a public health issue. The author argues that information, education, research and appropriate legislation and policies are essential components for effective anti-doping actions.

Ivan Waddington examines several social science approaches to understanding drug use in sport, including (1) social psychological game models; (2) drug use as a response to the biographical risks involved in athletic careers; (3) drug use as "overconformity" by athletes to the success goals of sport; and (4) medical sociological approaches which focus on the key relationship between athletes and sports physicians/team doctors.

Nader Ahmadi and **Göran Svedsäter** highlight, in Chapter 3, "The winner takes it all," the mechanisms underlying misuse of doping substances in society. They pose the question of how to explain and understand the phenomenon of doping and society, describing differences and similarities between doping in society and doping in sport. The authors highlight the problem of doping in a societal context and communicate relevant knowledge in relation to a sociological perspective, where doping is assumed to be a symptom of a social development. In the aftermath of the 1960s–1970s, where a large number of societies and individuals were swept by a wave of solidarity, returning to their roots/nature, and a general radicalization, the last few decades have witnessed a shift towards extreme forms of individualism with an emphasis on individual success, happiness and well-being.

David Hoff discusses the differences and similarities between doping in sport and doping in society by exploring theoretical and empirical explanations of doping use outside the sport context. The author's focus is on the driving forces and motives for the use of different doping preparations, and on the physiological and social consequences. This chapter includes discussions on the relationship between doping in society and risk, substance abuse and doping; the body ideals of society; the medicalization of society; doping in an individualized society; and, ideals of performance.

Hans Geyer describes how, in recent years, two new sources of doping substances for the fitness and recreational sports enthusiast have been established: the market for adulterated nutritional supplements and the market for unapproved pharmaceuticals. In the market for adulterated nutritional supplements, products containing undeclared stimulants, anabolic steroids and ß2-agonists have been detected. All these compounds are doping substances, available only, if at all, on prescription. These adulterated supplements are advertised as having the effects of the undeclared doping agents such as fat loss, muscle growth and increased training motivation. The doping substances are mixed into the nutritional supplements in therapeutic or even supra-therapeutic doses and are connected with severe health risks. Therefore medical doctors treating inexplicable health problems in fitness enthusiasts and recreational athletes should also take into consideration that these health problems may be due to the unintentional consumption of doping substances via nutritional supplements. The author also illuminates the black market of unapproved pharmaceuticals still in pre-clinical or clinical trials, which seems also to be a growing source of doping substances for fitness enthusiasts and recreational athletes. The growing number of internet providers for unapproved substances indicates an increasing demand.

Letizia Paoli discusses some of the findings of a study on the doping market in Italy, carried out by the author together with Alessandro Donati on behalf of the World Anti-Doping Agency. This study attempted to single out the main characteristics of the illegal suppliers of doping products in Italy and develop a typology of them based on their profession or occupation. The author also focuses on a special category of actors, officials of national sports bodies, including in this both the Italian National Olympic Committee (CONI) and sports federations. On the basis of this analysis, she concludes that the market for doping products is a peculiar semi-illegal one that, in its elite section, has long enjoyed the protection, if not the tolerance, of government representatives.

Clément de Maillard and **Elena Titova** describe the framework of a partnership with the World Anti-Doping Agency (WADA), and how the International Criminal Police Organization INTERPOL is dealing with both the doping of athletes in sport and the trafficking of performance-enhancing drugs destined for mass consumption. In this second field, INTERPOL's anti-doping project has developed an innovative approach. Driven by an intelligence-led approach, the anti-doping project defined its plan in terms of three steps. The first step was the definition of the issue: from a police perspective, it appeared essential to define precisely what is meant by performance-enhancing drugs (PED). Then, the second step was to watch the PED black market in order to determine its mechanisms, its specificities and the relationships between stakeholders (consumers, suppliers, producers, etc.). The last step consisted in building an ad hoc strategy. The authors also describe a case study on the re-emergence of 2,4-dinitrophenol.

Sigmund Loland and **Michael J. McNamee** critically examine the rationale for anti-doping. Their point of departure is WADA's normative criterion of "the spirit of sport." More specifically, a detailed and updated interpretation is proposed of "the spirit of sport." The interpretation includes considerations of fairness and justice in sport as well as of the health and welfare of athletes. It is argued that a detailed interpretation of "the spirit of sport" can be of help in line-drawing when it comes to distinguishing between acceptable and non-acceptable performance-enhancing biotechnologies. Moreover, it is argued that the interpretation can serve as a full-bodied justification of anti-doping in sport. This is considered to be of key importance in a situation with significant development and increased use of various performance-enhancing biotechnologies in many areas of life.

The authors chart the history of the idea of "the spirit of sport," especially in relation to anti-doping policy. They critically examine the idea of the three criteria for inclusion on WADA's Prohibited List from a philosophical perspective, drawing on arguments from conceptual analysis and conceptual vagueness. They then offer a defense of the "spirit of sport" argument as a means (1) to counter the individualized medicalization of doping and (2) to give normative force to anti-doping policy and education. Their conclusion is that, insofar as doping is to be considered a public health issue, a broader perspective is required that moves away from an exclusive focus on elite sports.

Tom Murray carries out a brief survey of the most important arguments offered by anti-doping sceptics in order to provide the background against which the case against doping in sport must be made. Further, he discusses that the ethical foundation of anti-doping rests on three principles: promote fairness; protect health: and preserve meaning. Fairness requires assuring that no athlete has an unfair advantage over his or her competitors. Anti-doping programs attempt to ensure fairness. Fairness, however, could also be achieved by allowing all athletes to use performance-enhancing technologies. His conclusion is that, along with protecting health, the justification for anti-doping rests on the meanings and values we find in it.

According to **Theodore Friedmann** sport is an important and deeply human activity. There are immense pressures on athletes to perform well, and athletes have responded historically to such pressure by devising multitudes of methods to gain competitive advantage over rivals. Friedman suggests that modern doping is the result of a balance between the efforts of those who seek to reduce or eliminate doping and those who respond by designing and implementing techniques and tools to evade restrictions on the use of the drugs and techniques of doping. He foresees that in the coming few years, will reflect the growing temptation to manipulate and "improve" normal human traits and the continuing struggle between forces that would permit, even encourage, all possible doping applications of science and those that wish to protect clean sport as a central human activity.

Pictures from the fight against doping in sport and society

WADA: public health work against doping in society

David Howman

WADA is the international independent organization created in 1999 to promote, coordinate and monitor the fight against doping in sport in all its forms. WADA's role is to protect the rights of clean athletes, and ensure their full confidence in the global anti-doping system.

In 2007, the cost of illicit drug use in the United States alone totaled more than $193 billion. Direct and indirect costs attributable to illicit drug use are estimated in three principal areas: crime, health and productivity. The buyers of these drugs are not exclusively elite athletes or their entourage. Today's doper has many faces. The emphasis on winning, record-setting and record-breaking fosters a "win at all costs," "look the other way" culture in which individuals will take extreme risks to achieve financial gain and personal glory.

Doping is no longer an issue confined to elite sport. It permeates other areas of our society, putting at risk individual and collective physical, mental and social well-being. Doping is not limited to elite sport. It has become a public health issue of such magnitude that, if unchecked, could reach pandemic proportions. Today's doper can be found in high schools and universities, among armed forces, at amateur sport competitions and in local gyms, and includes those young and old who seek to improve their physical appearance. Proactive, coordinated action is required to effectively address the scourge of doping globally on all fronts – through awareness, education and comprehensive legislation, and by leveraging information, expertise, alliances and partnerships across regulating bodies, industries and geographies. Young men and women are doping to improve their physique, while older generations seek the illusive "fountain of youth." Use of appearance- and performance-enhancing drugs (APEDS) is widespread.

Predominant substances and methods traded in the black market include:

- blood manipulations
- anabolic steroids and modulators
- hormones and hormonal modulators
- gene doping.

We must confront complacency and ensure there is long-term commitment from all. A proper mix of prevention and deterrence, and greater regard by our youth for values, will result in a more level playing field. Further alliances with the pharmaceutical industry and the arms of government, such as health, along with recognition of the fact that doping is not limited to elite athletes, will be of benefit to our young people and society in general.

Those who play down the social and behavioral dangers of doping underestimate the extent of its corrosive nature and destructive influence. Too often, government and industry either turn a blind eye or are implicit benefactors from the spoils of doping. The other side of that coin – society pays the high price for health care and rehabilitation for the ills of individuals that are seriously affected by the use of prohibited substances. Proactive, coordinated action is required to effectively address the scourge of doping globally on all fronts – through awareness, education and strong legislation, and by leveraging expertise, alliances and partnerships across regulating bodies, industries and geographies.

Public health constituents can borrow from anti-doping's Big Five playbook to:

- build a global network that includes educators, coaches, health care professionals, sport and industry associations, law enforcement, governments, and other interested stakeholder bodies;
- create and share education and awareness programs, model guidelines, tool kits, and other resources;
- promote professional and institutional ethics and morals through universal codes, standards and practices;
- put consistent, effective anti-doping laws, regulations and sanctions in place as deterrents;
- fund pertinent research;
- cooperate with and contribute to anti-doping investigations.

By working together to fight doping, government, industry and the anti-doping community can positively influence ethics and moral values, and put measures in place that encourage organizations and individuals to make informed, healthy choices.

INTERPOL: the complex fight against the trafficking of doping substances

Mathieu Holz

INTERPOL is the world's largest international police organization, with 190 member countries and has four strategic priorities: (1) provide a secure global police communications network for connecting the National Central Bureau with national law enforcement agencies for all 190 member countries; (2) provide around-the-clock support to policing; (3) provide training to build crime-fighting capacity; and (4) assist in the identification of crime trends and criminal behavior.

Each INTERPOL member country maintains a National Central Bureau (NCB) staffed by national law enforcement officers. The role of an NCB is to participate in all of INTERPOL's activities, providing constant and active cooperation.

The cooperation agreement signed in 2009 between WADA and INTERPOL aims to enhance international cooperation and strengthen the exchange of operational data. This cooperation agreement is the first of its kind signed between the world largest police organization and an international independent agency and focusing on a dedicated and very complex issue.

The agreement between WADA and INTERPOL is the outcome of two motivating factors: there is a need for better coordination in the fight against doping, specifically the trafficking of doping substances by organized crime groups, and furthermore, WADA recognized the importance of cooperation with INTERPOL to facilitate the exchange of doping information.

The main objectives of this cooperation agreement are:

- Establish a framework for cooperation; facilitate the exchange of expertise along with the prevention and suppression of doping and trafficking in doping.
- Support enforcement of national and international anti-doping measures.
- Cooperate in the collection, storage and exchange of information.
- Arrange information sessions and seminars to raise awareness about the trafficking of doping substances.

INTERPOL supports member countries facing complex doping investigations with international connections. This support includes, but is not limited to, the following:

- Create a network of "Points of Contact" (POCs) within relevant international law enforcement agencies specializing in the fight against doping.

- In conjunction with WADA's Science Department and/or WADA's expert groups, provide technical and scientific support to criminal investigations, lead or coordinate international investigations (on request), arrange ad hoc working group meetings, liaise with the World Customs Organization to enhance customs cooperation and enforcement-related activities.
- Facilitate the exchange of operational data among INTERPOL member countries.
- Inform INTERPOL member countries and WADA about new doping substances and trends discovered during investigations.

INTERPOL is providing technical tools and advice for law enforcement and more particularly field officers involved with doping investigations. In this regard, the INTERPOL anti-doping project has established a criminal intelligence initiative dedicated to performance-enhancing drugs (PEDs) and asked INTERPOL member countries to share information regarding seizures. The main objective is to offer an operational and applicable analysis for law enforcement and to support them for domestic investigations with international links. In order to collect enough data, the anti-doping project manager requests pictures of the seized products, the chemical composition of seized products and the circumstances in which it was seized.

*WHO: public impact of doping**

Timothy Armstrong and Nicolas Clark
World Health Organization, Geneva

The World Health Organization (WHO) is the United Nations specialized agency for health. WHO was established in 1948 and comprises 194 member countries. Its mandated role is in:

- providing leadership *on matters critical to health and engaging in partnerships where joint action is needed*;
- *shaping the* research agenda *and stimulating the generation, translation and dissemination of valuable knowledge*;
- *setting* norms and standards *and promoting and monitoring their implementation*;
- *articulating* ethical and evidence-based *policy options*;
- *providing* technical support, *catalyzing change, and building sustainable institutional capacity*; and
- monitoring *the health situation and assessing health trends.*

 The authors are staff members of the World Health Organization. The authors alone are responsible for the views expressed in this publication and they do not necessarily represent the views, decisions or policies of the World Health Organization.

WHO's current priorities for global health action are to strengthen health systems, to promote health throughout the life-course, to prevent and control noncommunicable diseases (NCD) and mental health conditions, to combat communicable diseases (such as HIV/AIDS, TB, malaria), and to increase capacity for the preparedness, surveillance and response to outbreaks such as Ebola and SARS.

As part of WHO's role in promoting health it has a major role to play in supporting countries in implementing policies which support the participation of people of all ages, and in particular children, in physical activity and sport without the use of drugs and other harmful legal and illicit substances. At the time of writing, WHO has no one particular mandate to address doping in sport or the population at large. However, the issue of "drugs in sport" is relevant to many areas of WHO's mandated work. WHO notes with some concern that the issue of "doping" is now not only occurring in elite sport, but that the prevalence of use of "doping" is increasing in the general population and in school-aged children and adolescents.

The negative impacts on physical and mental health along with the negative social aspects of doping are well documented – participation in "drug-free" physical activity and sport is a central component to WHO's approach to preventing NCDs (such as heart disease, cancer, diabetes, lung disease), promoting mental health (such as reducing depression, stress, anxiety), reducing the risk of interpersonal violence, promoting safe and healthy schools and workplaces, and reducing risk of infections such as HIV/AIDS and hepatitis, among others. WHO has several partners for its implementation of programs relevant to preventing substance abuse in physical activity, sports, schools and workplaces – these include, but are not limited to, formal relationships with UNESCO for the delivery of quality physical education and drug-free sport, UNEP to promote safe facilities for physical activity and recreation, the International Olympic Committee (IOC) on the promotion of sport, physical activity and healthy lifestyle, and informal associations with WADA and other global and national entities which together are addressing the scourge of drugs in sport and physical activity.

In addition to the challenges doping presents to the fairness of competitive sport, the use of performance-enhancing substances and methods present significant health risks. The most commonly detected class of performance-enhancing substances – anabolic androgenic steroids (AAS), which account for approximately 50 percent of all doping – have a range of dose-related adverse effects, many of which can be fatal. Beyond the health effects, an additional concern with steroid use is the risk of aggressive violent behavior. Male steroid users have been found to exhibit more violence towards their female partners when taking steroids than when not taking steroids and compared to non-steroid-using controls.

There have been several attempts to measure the rates of harmful steroid use and dependence in different settings. Steroid dependence is defined as a pattern of use whereby the user continues use despite negative consequences; users lose the capacity to control their use, and instead their lives revolve more and more around steroid use. It is estimated that up to one million adolescents in the US alone may have been steroid-dependent at some time in their lives. The frequency and severity of adverse consequences of steroid use relates to the quantity and frequency of steroids consumed. It is clear that steroids are being consumed in quantities high enough to cause harm by a significant proportion of adolescents and gym users in many countries.

This combination of factors has led some to argue that doping, in particular AAS use, is no longer an issue which affects only selected elite athletes. It is becoming an issue of public health significance, especially and most worryingly among those who are our future – our children.

1 Doping and public health

Historical background

Arne Ljungqvist

Introduction

The use of chemical substances and compounds for the purpose of making the human mind and body feel better and/or perform better can be traced back thousands of years. One common example found in sports literature is the use of Ma Huang in China more than 5,000 years ago. It was an extract obtained from dried herbal plants of the Ephedra family which was used for its stimulating effects. Not until 1885 was the active component of Ma Huang isolated. Under the name of Ephedrine it came into use as an anti-asthmatic medication following further identification of its properties in the 1920s. It is a so-called "sympathicomimetic" substance, which means that it mimics the actions of the sympathetic nervous system by, for example, relaxing the smooth muscles of the respiratory tract. In addition, the substance can have a psychostimulating effect similar to amphetamine, although weaker. That effect made it appear together with amphetamine and other stimulants already on the first list of banned substances in sport that was decided upon by the International Olympic Committee (IOC) in 1967, the so-called "Prohibited List." Since then, the list has developed to include a large number of different substances and methods that have come into use in sport for the purpose of performance enhancement.

In 1999 the World Anti-Doping Agency (WADA) was created jointly by the IOC and the governments around the world, primarily for the establishment of a common set of doping rules that could be recognized by the sporting world and by the political and juridical establishments, the so-called WADA Code. In 2004 WADA took over the responsibility for the prohibited list from the IOC and incorporated it into the Code as an "International Standard." The list is updated every year. Many of the substances and methods that are on the prohibited list today have side effects, some perhaps not so important but others quite harmful. Furthermore, the use of some of the listed substances has spread outside the sports community, particularly to young people for whom sports stars are role models. The use of doping substances and methods is, therefore, becoming an increasingly important public health issue. In order to understand this evolution it is important to look back at the development of the prohibited list.

The development of the prohibited list

The 1967 IOC list was developed by the IOC Medical Commission (IOCMC) which was founded in 1961 following the death of a Danish cyclist during the team road race at the Rome Olympic Games the year before. He and some of his team mates had reportedly been given some stimulating drugs and the IOCMC was asked to design a strategy to combat the use of drugs in Olympic sport. Before then not much in the way of organized anti-doping activities had taken place in sport. True, the International Association of Athletics Federations (IAAF) was the first sports organization to introduce rules against the use of stimulants in athletics in 1928, but there are no reports from that time of any rule enforcement or doping controls. The IOCMC, therefore, started more or less from scratch, and it took the Commission six years to come up with an anti-doping strategy. It included a prohibited list and a proposal to conduct controls for the listed substances on Olympic participants.

The 1967 list included a number of classes of drugs that were known to be used by athletes for temporary performance enhancement [1]. They were (1) sympathicomimetic amines (including ephedrine), amphetamine and similar substances; (2) stimulants of the central nervous system (strychnine) and analeptics; (3) analgesic narcotics (e.g., morphine) and similar substances; (4) antidepressants (e.g., monoamine oxidase inhibitors), imipramine and similar substances; (5) major tranquillizers (e.g., phenothiazine).

The strategy developed by the IOC was introduced at the Olympic Games in 1968, although on a small scale. The first Olympic doping case occurred at the Summer Games in Mexico City when a member of the Swedish team in modern pentathlon tested positive for alcohol. The substance had been added to the IOC list explicitly for the shooting event in modern pentathlon and, ironically, on Swedish initiative. The athlete concerned was disqualified, and so was the Swedish team, which lost its bronze medal.

The Olympic Summer Games in Munich in 1972 was the first big sport event at which a large-scale doping control program was put in place. More than 2,000 samples were collected from the 7,121 athletes that participated. By then the list had been modified to include (1) psychomotor stimulants; (2) sympathicomimetic amines; (3) various stimulants acting on the central nervous system; (4) analgesic narcotics. It was noted that the list was not restrictive. A famous doping case occurred. The 16-year-old US swimmer Rick DeMont tested positive for ephedrine after he had won the gold medal in 400 meter freestyle. He had also qualified for the final in 1,500 meters, where he was the favorite to win another gold. Shortly before that final, however, his positive sample was reported by the laboratory, following which he was barred from the 1,500 meter final and also lost his gold medal in 400 meters. He had reported the use of ephedrine for his asthma but that was not considered as an excuse. There were no rules in place at that time for granting therapeutic use exemption.

It is noticeable that anabolic androgenic steroids (AAS) did not appear on the IOC list until 1976 despite the fact that such drugs were known to have been in use for at least 20 years [2] and that proof of their use at the Olympic Games was obtained in Mexico City in 1968 [3]. The philosophy of the IOC was not to ban substances for which there were no detection methods available. In 1974 the International Association of Athletics Federations banned the steroids and analyzed for them at the European Athletic Championships in Rome the same year using an immunologically based method. No positive cases were found but the initiative made the IOC add steroids to the list for the 1976 Olympic Summer Games at which eight cases were identified with an improved method.

At the 1984 Los Angeles Olympic Games the gold medal-winning US cycling team admitted that they had used blood transfusion in order to enhance their endurance, a method that was not banned at the time in the absence of a detection method. The admittance, however, made the IOC change philosophy. Blood doping (e.g., transfusion) was added to the list, and from then on substances and methods regarded as doping were added irrespective of the presence of detection methods. This made the list expand considerably during the decades that followed.

In 1998 it became known that an American baseball star was using a food supplement called Andro, which resulted in a boom for it on the sales market [4]. It turned out that Andro was actually androstendione, the immediate precursor of testosterone in the body and not banned at the time. However, the IOC placed androstendione on the prohibited list the same year, together with a number of other endogenous steroids. From then on the banned steroids have appeared on the list in two categories, one endogenous and one exogenous.

The main trigger for adding a substance to the list was reports that it was used by athletes for performance enhancement. Less frequently, additions were made on the basis of a scientific evaluation of the potentially performance enhancing effects of a newly developed drug. Today, however, WADA is cooperating with the pharmaceutical industry in order to have detection methods available for substances under development that may be misused for doping once they come on the market. To that effect, a new class of "non-approved substances" was recently added to the banned list and includes

> Any pharmacological substance which is not addressed by any of the subsequent sections on the List and with no current approval by any governmental regulatory health authority for human therapeutic use (e.g., drugs under pre-clinical or clinical development or discontinued, designer drugs, substances approved only for veterinary use) [5].

The general perception of "doping" is an illegal use of performance enhancing drugs or methods. The ambition to steadily have the list updated forces sport authorities to introduce new substances to the list as soon as their potential use for performance enhancement is suspected. To actually prove a performance enhancing effect would take years, if it was at all possible from ethical and legal points of view since athletes who dope take doses far above the therapeutic levels.

To solve the problem the WADA Code states that two out of the following three criteria should be satisfied for considering the inclusion of a new substance or method in the list, namely, that the substance/method can be judged to be (1) performance enhancing and/or (2) dangerous to the health and/or (3) against the spirit of sport. This means that a banned substance or method does not necessarily need to be performance enhancing. In practice, however, the potential performance enhancing effect of a substance or method is always taken into account when its inclusion in the list is considered, but the performance enhancing effect does not need to be proven.

During the IOC time (1967–2003) the list was decided upon by the IOCMC without any consultation process. Interestingly, the sports society did not ask for any. When WADA took over the responsibility for the list in 2004, however, a wide consultation process was inaugurated which includes all stakeholders such as the National Anti-Doping Organizations (NADOs), the International Federations (IFs), the IOC and others. This is an annual process during which WADA receives hundreds of submissions from stakeholders for consideration. On September 30 each year, the prohibited list for the following year is published on the WADA website.

The prohibited list is produced for the prevention of cheating in sport by using performance enhancing drugs that may also include clear health risks. It should be seen as a means to protect (1) athletes' health and (2) the integrity of sport by establishing as level a playing field as possible. However, some of the listed drugs have come into use in the general society outside sport. Particular concern has arisen about the wide non-medical use of AAS in the younger generation, since such use can be quite harmful. While the dangerous stimulants on the list are mostly covered by appropriate legislation (e.g., anti-narcotic laws), such legislation against AAS exists in only a few countries [6]. This is all the more deplorable as the misuse of AAS among young people for other purposes than success in sport has long been known [7, 8].

What are AAS and why are they used?

AAS are derivatives of the male sex hormone testosterone the endogenous production of which increases during puberty in males. Its effects on the body can roughly be divided into an "androgenic" effect and an "anabolic" effect. The androgenic effect includes the development of the typical male secondary sex characteristics such as the enlargement of penis and testes, the male body hair distribution and deepening of the voice. It also has an effect on behavioral features including aggression, which could possibly also be regarded as an androgenic effect. The typical anabolic effects are the result of a promotion of protein synthesis and include growth and strengthening of tissues such as muscles, connective tissue and bone.

Following the isolation of testosterone in 1935 and the identification of its biological properties, attempts were made to synthesize chemical derivatives of the testosterone molecule with a minimum of androgenic and a maximum of anabolic effect. Such substances would be particular useful in the treatment of women with tissue-devastating diseases. Such drugs came to be known as just "anabolic steroids" and found their way into sport in the late 1950s/early 1960s because of their muscle-building properties.

AAS use in sport

It was at the World Games in Moscow in 1956 that a physician in the US team, John B. Ziegler, witnessed the use of testosterone by Soviet athletes [2]. In an attempt to give US athletes similar opportunities to perform well Dr Ziegler approached the CIBA pharmaceutical company after his return home and helped them produce an anabolic steroid with muscle-building effects and reduced androgenic effects. It was given the name Dianabol and, although the androgen effect turned out to be quite significant, it became the fashion steroid in sport far into the 1970s and beyond [9]. The East Germans produced their own anabolic steroid named Oral Turinabol, which was systematically used in their state-run doping regime until German reunification in 1990 [10].

Once AAS became banned in sport there were no longer any possibilities to conduct properly designed scientific studies in order to elucidate their believed performance enhancing effects in different sports, nor their side effects, particularly since athletes were taking the substances in dosages far above the therapeutic norms. During the late 1970s and throughout the 1980s an intense debate took place about the effects of AAS. In the absence of clear scientific data practical experience played a significant role. In general, athletes strongly believed in the performance enhancing effects and were inclined to disregard, or even deny, their side effects. After the Canadian sprinter Ben Johnson tested positive for AAS (stanozolol) at the 1988 Seoul Olympic Games, the Canadian government arranged a thorough inquiry led by Ontario chief justice Charles Dubin, at which the author of this article was heard as witness. In his final report in 1990 Dubin concluded that "The overwhelming evidence of this inquiry is that anabolic steroids enhance athletic performance" [11]. This is strongly supported by the experience of the East German doping program [10]. Today, no one doubts the performance enhancing effects of AAS, which for many years have made up between 50 and 60 percent of the doping cases in sport.

The use of AAS for doping and the fight against that use have their own history which has been described in a large number of publications [e.g., 12, 13, 14, 15]. Their use outside sport, on the other hand, has received less attention, and there has been little opposition to that use.

AAS use outside sport

The muscle-building effects of AAS was picked up by people practicing "body building" [e.g., 16, 17], which is a recognized sport in some countries but not in others. The use also spread to other young people who were interested in neither competitive sport nor body building as such, but who were unhappy with their own body image. In this way the AAS found their way into gyms and fitness centers and came to be used as a muscle-building fashion drug by adolescents around the world from the 1980s or earlier [e.g., 18, 19, 20, 21, 22, 23, 24]. Although most users were found to be boys and young men, girls and young women were not exempted. In the late 1980s about 6.6 percent of male high school students in a range of states in the US were using AAS [8], and in a Swedish study published some ten years later, 3.6 percent of the 16-year-old and 2.8 percent of the 17-year-old high school boys reported AAS misuse [25]. There is evidence also that those who use AAS for body image reasons take them in dosages far above therapeutic levels, just like athletes [26].

In a recently published European survey including Denmark, the Netherlands, Sweden, Poland and Cyprus [27], it was suggested that 1–2 percent of the population in the participating countries currently use or have experience with the use of AAS or other performance and image enhancing drugs (PIEDs), which means between 700,000 and 1.4 million people. The users are usually young and middle-aged men, most of whom take the substances for body image reasons. It was also found that the steroid users are over-represented among fitness center members compared with the population in general. It was concluded that "the use of steroids and other performance and image enhancing drugs (PIEDs) is a current problem in society."

Health risks associated with AAS abuse

Most of the drugs on the prohibited list are medications which are intended for use on medical indications and for which harmful side effects of therapeutic dosages are well known. When used for the purpose of doping, however, athletes tend to believe that the more you take the more doping effects will you get. This is particularly true for anabolic androgenic steroids which has been by far the most used group of doping substances for several decades.

As mentioned above, the side effects of high dosages of AAS are virtually impossible to assess scientifically, since studies using the appropriate scientific protocols cannot be conducted. However, conclusions can be drawn from what is known about the biological action of AAS, the side effects of the use in therapeutic dosages and the massive experience there is today from the use of AAS in sport for the past 50 years or more.

Early recorded effects of therapeutic use of AAS were the retardation and stopping of growth when given to children and adolescents due to premature closing of the epiphyseal growth zones in the long bones and, although rarely, the development of abnormal blood vessels in the liver (peliosis hepatis) that could give rise to dangerous bleedings. The additional health risks associated with AAS abuse can roughly be ascribed to the anabolic and/or androgenic/endocrinological and even toxic actions on organs and functions of the body. In their review Buettner and Thieme [28] listed "Possible adverse effects of AAS abuse."[1]

The organ damage and symptoms could certainly be the result of other factors than abuse of AAS. On the other hand, users of AAS seem to run particular risks in developing the mentioned damages to the cardiovascular and musculoskeletal systems, the liver and the skin. The same is also true for the male- and female-specific effects. In addition, the psycho-behavioral disturbances have received particular attention. It would seem that AAS abuse may, indeed, lead to aggressive actions beyond the person's control, including violent crime, but that it would occur only in persons with a particular personality [29]. The same is probably true for those who develop dependence and depressive symptoms, which may result in suicide [30].

Public health aspects and concerns

The spread of the use of doping substances, particularly AAS, outside sport as described above slowly became a concern for public authorities. In Sweden, for example, a governmental inquiry was launched in the late 1980s. Customs data showed that there was a considerable illegal import of AAS that could not possibly be explained by a use limited to elite sport in the country. Legislation was found to be necessary but existing laws relating to narcotics and medications were judged to be inadequate for the purpose. A new law against certain doping substances (including AAS) was created, which criminalized unauthorized production, possession and trafficking of those substances. It came into force on July 1, 1992. In 1999 the law was amended to include criminalization also of consumption of doping substances such as AAS. However, only a few countries have taken similar actions [6] despite the fact that the use of AAS in society in general has been increasingly recognized as a public health issue and that negative health effects are probably underreported by the medical community [31].

The extensive use of so-called "food supplements" or "dietary supplements" in today's society is a further cause of concern. The production and sales of such supplements are not subjected to the same strict regulations and supervision as genuine medications and it is not unusual for them to contain proscribed substances, including AAS [32, 33]. Furthermore, there is an aggressive and sometimes misleading marketing of the supplements and they are easily available on the internet, as are AAS [34]. This means an obvious risk of athletes testing positive inadvertently [35] and keeps the door wide open for steroid misuse in society.

In order to place the public health aspect of the use of doping substances on the agenda, an international symposium on "Doping as a public health issue" was organized in Stockholm in September 2012 by the Professor Arne Ljungqvist Anti-Doping Foundation. For the first time representatives from the relevant international organizations, i.e., WADA, the IOC, WHO, UNESCO and INTERPOL, came together and addressed the issue, together with over 100 experts from various fields around the world.

At the end of the symposium a statement was worked out *in plenum* [36]. It should be noted, however, that the participants had not been asked to bring along any authorization to sign a final agreement on behalf of their organizations. The statement was, therefore, signed by the Chairman of the organizing Foundation. It contained the following basic elements:

1. The misuse of doping substances in the broader society has to be clearly differentiated from doping in elite sport and, to some degree, also from doping in recreational sport as their motives differ. However, elite athletes can be used as role models for all young people.
2. The increased misuse of doping substances and the use of nutritional supplements is part of the modern society and needs to be approached not only as an individual problem but as a societal issue.
3. The ideals of health and fitness in today's society have to be understood and dissected since the health ideals, paradoxically, could lead to increased use of doping substances in the quest for better physical performance, appearance and/or self-esteem.
4. The misuse of doping substances in the broader society must be analyzed from a multidisciplinary approach that includes issues of ethics, human health, environmental and social sciences.
5. In spite of the serious nature of the doping problem, there is limited knowledge about the underlying causes of doping. Additional research in this area will contribute to the development of improved strategies and choices of preventive measures. The results of such research should be collected at a global level, e.g., in a database such as the one UNESCO has created.
6. From public health and sports perspective, information, education, research and appropriate legislation and policies are essential components for effective anti-doping actions.
7. The misuse of doping substances in the broader society is a health and security issue. Action must be taken by governments and organizations within a harmonized international legal framework and policies.
8. Transparency, harmonization, information sharing, greater intelligence gathering efforts and more efficient use of existing resources, including media, amongst all partners on a global level involved in the fight against doping, are essential.
9. Law enforcement agencies and sport organizations should work together to enforce existing laws and to deter and bring to justice illegal manufacturers, traffickers and suppliers of doping substances.
10. Governments have responsibilities to protect their citizens from misusing doping substances by providing information and education about the dangers of such misuse.
11. Yet, governments cannot solve the problem by themselves. Individuals have a role to play in their own behaviors and decisions in the anti-doping effort. It is all about integrity, dignity and honor.

Conclusions

Doping is the use in sport of substances and methods that appear on the so-called "prohibited list."

From its inception in the 1960s up to and including 2003, the list was decided upon by the IOC and from then on by WADA.

The list has evolved over time from first having included only stimulants, via the inclusion of AAS in the 1970s, to the comprehensive list of today which includes a large number of modern therapeutic drugs and methods, e.g., gene therapy.

Many listed substances have long been used outside sport, such as amphetamines and cocaine, the use of which is regulated by legislation.

The use of AAS outside sport has become a particular concern to society since it seems to be increasing, entails significant health risks and lacks specific legislation in most countries.

Today, the use of AAS outside sport is recognized as a public health issue that needs to be addressed by governments through information, education, research and appropriate legislation.

Note

1 *Cardiovascular system:* Disturbed lipid metabolism, elevated blood pressure – hypertension, myocardial hypertrophy, cardiac arrhythmias, cardiomyopathy, thrombosis, early myocardial infarction, sudden death; *Endocrine/reproductive system:* Decrease of libido and fertility, decreased LH and FSH, altered glucose metabolism; *Male specific effects*: Testicular atrophy, erectile dysfunction and impotence, subfertility, prostatic hypertrophy, impaired spermatogenesis, gynecomastia (hypertrophy of the breast glands); *Female specific effects:* Virilization, voice deepening, menstrual irregularities, clitoral enlargement, breast atrophy; *Liver:* Cholestasis and jaundice, peliosis hepatis, tumor development, gall bladder stones; *Psycho-behavioral disturbances:* Mood swings, aggressiveness, depressive and or manic symptoms, sleep disturbances, dependence with withdrawal symptoms, psychosis; *Kidney:* Pollakisuria, increase of serum creatinine, kidney stones; *Skin.* Acne, urticaria, striae, alopecia; *Gastrointestinal tract:.* Queasiness, emesis, diarrhea, hematemesis; *Musculoskeletal:* Tendon damage, bone pain, premature epiphyseal closure (adolescents); *Various:* Edema, fever and shivers, anaphylactic shock, injection-related effects such as infection, hematoma and hepatitis B or C and HIV infection.

References

1 Dirix, A. and Sturbois, X., *The First Thirty Years of the International Olympic Committee Medical Commission 1967–1997.* 1998; IOC Olympic Study Centre, Lausanne.
2 Voy, R., *Drugs, Sport and Politics.* 1991; Leisure Press, Champaign, IL.
3 Buhre, B., Hormoninjektion utan dopingutslag. In Pettersson, S.-U. (ed.) *Olympiaboken 1968.* 1969; Brunnhages Förlag AB, Stockholm, p. 104.
4 Catlin, D.H., Fitch, K.D. and Ljungqvist, A., Medicine and science in the fight against doping in sport. *J. Int. Med.* 2008; 264:99–114.
5 The Prohibited List 2015. www.wada-ama.org.
6 Houlihan, B. and García, B., *The Use of Legislation to Controlling the Production, Movement, Importation, Distribution and Supply of Performance Enhancing Drugs in Sport (PEDS).* www.wada-ama.org/en/media/news/2012-11/loughborough-study-supports-doping-specific-legislation. Accessed November 15, 2012.
7 Corder, B.W., Dezelsky, T.L., Toohey, J.V. and Di Vito, C.L., An analysis of trends in drug use behavior at five American universities. *J. Sch. Health* 1974; 44:386–389.
8 Buckley, W.E., Yesalis, C.E., Friedl, K.E., Anderson, W.A., Streit, A.L. and Wright,

J.E., Estimated prevalence of anabolic steroids among male high school seniors. *JAMA* 1988; 260:3441–3445.
9 Sinner, D. and Bachmann, M., *Das Schwarze Buch.* 2004; BMS Verlag, Gronau, pp. 239–270.
10 Berendonk, B., *Doping Dokumente – von der Forschung zum Betrug.* 1991; Springer, Berlin-Heidelberg.
11 Dubin, Ch.L., *Commission of Inquiry into the Use of Drugs and Banned Practices Intended to Increase Athletic Performance.* 1990; Canadian Government Publishing Centre, Ottawa, p. 103.
12 Houlihan, B., *Dying to Win*, second edn. 2002; Council of Europe Publishing, Strasbourg.
13 Thieme, D. and Hemmersbach, P. (eds), *Doping in Sports.* 2010; Springer, Heidelberg.
14 Lager, G., *Doping's Nemesis.* 2011; Sports Books, Cheltenham.
15 Paoli, L. and Donati, A., *The Sports Doping Market – Understanding Supply and Demand, and the Challenges of Their Control.* 2014; Springer, New York.
16 Lindström, M., Nilsson, A., Katzman, P.L., Manzon, L. and Dymling, J.F., Use of anabolic–androgenic steroids in body builders – frequency and attitudes. *J. Int. Med.* 1990; 227:407–411.
17 Delbeke, F.T., Desmet, M. and Debackere, M., The abuse of doping agents in competing body builders in Flanders (1988–1993). *Int. J. Sports Med.* 1995; 16:66–70.
18 Handelsman, D.J. and Gupta, L., Prevalence and risk factors for anabolic–androgenic steroid abuse in Australian high school students. *Int. J. Androl.* 1997; 20:159–164.
19 DuRant, R.H., Escobedo, L.G. and Heath, G.W., Anabolic steroid use, strength training and multiple drug use among adolescents in the United States. *Pediatrics* 1995; 96:23–28.
20 Williamson, D.J., Anabolic steroid use among students in a British college of technology. *Br. J. Sport Med.* 1993; 27:200–201.
21 Nilsson, S., Androgenic anabolic steroid use among male adolescents in Falkenberg. *Eur. J. Clin. Pharmacol.* 1995; 48:9–11.
22 Lambert, M.I., Titlestad, S.D. and Schwellnus, M.P., Prevalence of androgenic-anabolic steroid use in adolescents in two regions of South Africa. *S. Afr. Med. J.* 1998; 88:876–880.
23 Melia, P., Pipe, A. and Greenberg, L., The use of anabolic-androgenic steroids by Canadian students. *Clin. J. Sport Med.* 1996; 6:9–14.
24 Maharaj, V.R., Dookie, T., Mohammed, S., Ince, S., Marsang, B.L., Rambocas, N., Chin, M., McDougall, L. and Teelucksingh, S., Knowledge, attitudes and practices of anabolic steroid usage among gym users in Trinidad. *West Indian Med. J.* 2000; 49:55–58.
25 Nilsson, S., Misuse of anabolic steroids in youth: trends, attitudes and evaluation of intervention programme. Academic thesis, 2003; Kompendiet AB, Gothenburg.
26 Parkinson, A.B. and Evans, N.A., Anabolic androgenic steroids: a survey of 500 users. *Med. Sci. Sports and Exerc.* 2006; 38:644–651.
27 Anti-Doping Denmark, *Strategy for Stopping Steroids*, first edn. 2012; Anti-Doping Denmark, Copenhagen.
28 Buettner, A. and Thieme, D., Side effects of anabolic androgenic steroids: pathological findings and structure–activity relationships. In Thieme, D. and Hemmersbach, P. (eds), *Doping in Sports.* 2010; Springer, Heidelberg.
29 Pope, H.G. Jr, Kougi, E.M. and Hudson, J.I., Effects of supraphysiologic doses of testosterone on mood an aggression in normal men: a randomized control trial. *Arch. Gen. Psychiatry* 2000; 57:133–140.

30 Thiblin, I., Runeson, B. and Rajs, J., Anabolic androgenic steroids and suicide. *Ann. Clin. Psychiatry* 1999; 11:223–231.

31 Sjöqvist, F., Garle, M. and Rane, A., Use of doping agents, particularly anabolic steroids, in sports and society. *Lancet* 2008; 371:1872–1882.

32 Geyer, H., Parr, M.K., Mareck, U., Reinhart, U., Schrader, Y. and Schänzer, W. Analysis of non-hormonal nutritional supplements for anabolic-androgenic steroids – results of an international study. *Int. J. Sports Med.* 2004; 25:124–129.

33 Abbate, V., Kicman, A.T., Evans-Brown, M., McVeigh, J., Cowan, D.A., Wilson, C., Coles, S.J. and Walker, C.J., Anabolic steroids detected in bodybuilding dietary supplements – a significant risk to public health. *Drug Test Anal.* 2014; October 6 doi: 10. 1002/dta. 1728 [Epub ahead of print].

34 Cordaro, F.G., Lombardo, S. and Consentino, M., Selling androgenic anabolic steroids by the pound: identification and analysis of popular websites on the internet. *Scand. J. Med. Sci. Sports* 2011; 21:247–259.

35 Geyer, H., Schänzer, W. and Thevis, M., Anabolic agents: recent strategies for their detection and protection from inadvertent doping. *Brit. J. Sports Med.* 2014; 48:820–826.

36 Professor Arne Ljungqvist Anti-Doping Foundation. http://arneljungqvist.com/news/94-1210-symposium-statement-published. Accessed October 22, 2012.

2 Social and behavioural science perspectives on drug use in sport

Ivan Waddington

Introduction

The key distinguishing characteristic of all social science perspectives on drug use in sport is that they seek to understand the behaviour of drug-using athletes not by focusing on the athlete as an individual, but by locating athletes within the network of relationships in which they are involved within sport. This typically involves a focus not just on the athletes' relationships with others in what Nixon (1992) has called the 'sportsnet', that is the web of interaction with other athletes, coaches, managers, team physicians and others, but also on broader social changes such as the increasing competitiveness and commercialization of sport.

The central objective of this chapter is to outline some of the major social and behavioural theories of drug use in sport, including: (1) differential association; (2) Marxist approaches; (3) drug use as 'overconformity' by athletes to the success goals of sport; (4) social psychological game models; (5) drug use as a response to the biographical risks involved in athletic careers; and (6) medical sociological approaches which focus on the key relationship between athletes and sports physicians/team doctors. It should be noted that these theories are not mutually exclusive and many share overlapping or similar ideas about how we can best understand drug use in sport.

Differential association

In two useful reviews of social scientific work on drug use in sport, Lüschen (1993, 2000) identified several theoretical approaches which, he suggested, could help in understanding the use of performance-enhancing drugs in sport. One of these was the theory of differential association which had originally been developed by Sutherland and Cressey (1974), not with a view to explaining drug use in sport but with a view to explaining deviant behaviour more generally within the wider society. Lüschen suggested that this approach could usefully be applied to understanding drug use in sport, not least because it indicates that the use of performance-enhancing drugs cannot be understood as the behaviour of isolated individuals, for the use of drugs implies not only a network of relationships between users and suppliers, but drug use itself is seen as a process involving learning from, and encouragement by, others such as peers and affiliates (Lüschen 1993, 2000). Both these, Lüschen suggests, indicate how the use of illicit drugs 'is performed as part of a deviant subculture, or by a group of persons that show features of secret societies' (2000: 466). In this context, the theory of differential association suggests that, in order to explain the use of drugs in sport we need to explore the particular subculture of drug-using athletes and suppliers of drugs, including the involvement of coaches, physicians and other members of what has been called the 'doping network' (Waddington and Smith 2009: 58). While Lüschen noted that this approach is 'mainly descriptive' – and in this regard it might be said that it is a loose theoretical framework, or perhaps a group of sensitizing concepts, rather than a theory proper – he also suggested that it nevertheless 'suggests quite a number of research questions and interpretive suggestions' (2000: 466). It might also be noted that a key premise of the theory of differential association – that drug use is a *socially learned* activity – has been incorporated into other theoretical approaches which have sought to identify the key patterns of association between athletes and others within 'doping networks'.

The importance of understanding the subculture of those involved in drug use is clearly brought out in Monaghan's (2001) study of steroid-using bodybuilders. Monaghan documents the popular negative stereotyping of bodybuilders as 'steroid freaks' subject to ' 'roid rage', but what is of particular interest are the bodybuilders' responses to, and their rejection of, these negative stereotypes. Monaghan counterposes what he calls 'mainstream' culture with the bodybuilders' subcultural understandings and background expectancies which, he says, enable them to 'normalize' and rationalize activities which others tend to consider as deviant, dangerous and risky. There is, he suggests, 'a general perception among bodybuilders that they inhabit a community under threat, leading many to engage in discursive stratagems to resist connotations of moral or social odium' (Monaghan 2001: 26). One such stratagem involves pointing to the deficiencies of 'bodybuilder' and 'bodybuilding' as descriptive labels while stressing that their pursuit should be conceived as a process of shaping, refining and sculpting the body rather than simply building size.

Also pertinent in this regard is a study of drug use in sport which was carried out by PMP Consultancy on behalf of the European Commission. PMP held discussions with two focus groups consisting of young national-level British athletes and a group of coaches at various levels from national team to local club. The data from these two focus groups shed some interesting light on whether athletes themselves regard drug use as deviant. Particularly striking was the fact that the coaches not only generally agreed that the incidence of illicit drug use in elite sport was high but – and this is of particular interest in the context of the commonly held view that drug use is a form of deviance – they also felt that the use of such drugs was considered acceptable within the community of elite athletes and that, *far from being considered deviant, the use of drugs was actually considered to represent conformity within elite athletics* (PMP Consultancy 2001: 32).

Other studies which similarly emphasize the need to understand the subculture in which drug-using athletes are involved include those by Waddington (2000) and Hoberman (2003) of what has been called the 'culture of tolerance' of doping in professional cycling, while the 'conspiracy of silence' among drug-using athletes – also known as the 'brotherhood of the needle' (Dubin 1990: 336) – also points to the need to understand the subculture of drug-using athletes. Perhaps above all what this approach suggests, and these studies confirm, is that one cannot adequately understand drug use in sport by focusing on the individual drug-using athlete, without reference to the wider network of relationships in which s/he is involved.

Marxist approaches

Lüschen (1993, 2000) has suggested that Marxist theory may also be useful in understanding aspects of drug use in sport. He noted that Marxist theory suggests that the use of drugs is indicative of the alienation of individuals – in this case athletes – in modern capitalist societies. Marxist sociologists, he suggests, could identify many structural clues that would illustrate 'how human beings have lost touch with their true nature, how the athlete as a controlled human being is exploited and alienated, or how sport itself produces alienation' (Lüschen 1993: 100). In this regard, Lüschen argues that such an approach would tend to emphasize that the 'objective situation of an athlete is more significant than what the athlete subjectively feels'; in this approach, he suggests, a recognition that drug-using athletes often knowingly and willingly engage in drug use 'would be irrelevant in such a framework' for it is the wider structure which generates alienation which is the focus of analysis (1993: 100). As Coakley (2007: 156) has noted, within this perspective athletes are viewed as 'victims of a profit-driven system'. It is certainly the case that Marxist writers on sport such as Brohm (1978) and Rigauer (1981) have argued that, under capitalism, elite-level athletes are simply new types of workers and that, as sport becomes just another form of work, so it comes to represent constraint rather than freedom, with the removal of all playful elements and creative spontaneity; within such a framework, drug use may be seen as a form of alienation of sports workers. For example, Brohm (1978: 19) has suggested that even a world record holder in athletics may be seen as 'a slave of the track', while drug use is seen as an aspect of alienation in sport, 'stemming from the oppression of the body pushed to the limits of physical effort' (Brohm 1978: 23).

In addition to the classic Marxist approaches of Brohm and Rigauer, elements of this approach can also be found in the work of writers such as Bryson. Bryson (1990) notes that the 'amateur ethos', with its emphasis on pursuit of the activity as an end in itself, norms of 'fair play' and a chivalrous attitude of friendly rivalry towards opponents, developed in a specific place and time – England in the nineteenth century – and she suggests that this 'historic amateur code' was 'never meant to support an emphasis on winning, and certainly not with the additional pressures that come with the current possibility of major financial rewards'

(Bryson 1990: 150). She suggests that, in contrast to the amateur code, the values of modern sport, and in particular the emphasis on winning, 'are more consonant with the values of modern capitalism and advanced industrialisation generally' and, in a conclusion which echoes the Marxist idea that sport can, and should, be a free, playful and non-alienating activity, she suggests that:

> if we were to aim to change the situation more than to merely keep drug use under some reasonable level of control, quite fundamental changes would be necessary. This would require a focus away from profit making and competition, towards the style of cooperative sport favoured by some feminists and critics of capitalism. While such a transformation may seem unlikely in the current circumstances it is a vision that needs to be nurtured by all who would like to see sport move closer to goals such as equality, personal development, democratic involvement and fun for all.
>
> (Bryson 1990: 151–152)

This approach therefore holds that the traditional values of 'fair play' have been systematically undermined by broader social processes which have impinged upon the development of sport since the late nineteenth century and that drug use is a more or less inevitable aspect of modern sport forms which embody the key values of modern capitalism and, in particular, the values of competition and commercialism.

Drug use as deviant overconformity

The American sociologist Jay Coakley offers a novel and interesting approach to understanding drug use in sport, and one which runs counter to many commonly held ideas about those who are sometimes emotively described as 'drug cheats' and who may be seen as people who simply disregard sporting values. Coakley suggests that, on the contrary, drug use in sport can be seen as a form of what he calls 'deviant overconformity' to key aspects of the sport ethic. He notes that explanations of deviance are often rooted in the idea of 'underconformity': that is, deviants do not conform to widely accepted standards of behaviour. As he puts it, this involves the idea that deviant behaviour, such as drug use, is 'based on ignoring or rejecting norms' (Coakley 2007: 159). However, he suggests that this is misleading, for drug use by athletes cannot be understood simply as a rejection of key sporting values; on the contrary, it expresses not only an acceptance of, but an *overconformity* to, key values within the sport ethic, most notably the value attached to winning which may lead athletes to use performance-enhancing drugs in their pursuit of sporting success. In this sense, drug use can be seen as a form of *deviant overconformity* based on 'uncritically accepting norms and being willing to follow them to extreme degrees' (Coakley 2007: 159). In this regard he suggests that research indicates that 'drug and substance use by athletes generally is not the result of defective socialization or lack of moral character because many users and abusers are the most dedicated, committed, and hard-working athletes in sports' (Coakle, 2007: 175–178); rather, he suggests:

> most substance use and abuse seems to be an expression of uncritical acceptance of the norms of the sport ethic. Therefore, it is grounded in overconformity – the same type of overconformity that occurs when injured distance runners continue training, even when training may cause serious injuries; when young female gymnasts control weight by cutting their food intake to dangerous levels; and when NFL players use painkilling drugs and risk their already injured and surgically repaired bodies week after painful week.
>
> (Coakley 2007: 178)

Coakley notes that not all athletes are equally likely to overconform to the sport ethic and he hypothesises that those most likely to do so would include athletes who have low self-esteem or are so eager to be accepted as athletes that they will do whatever it takes to be acknowledged by their peers in sport, and athletes who see achievement in sports as the only way to get ahead and gain respect.

Game models: the social psychology of drug use

In the game models approach, doping is seen as a 'game' in which athletes decide to use or not to use drugs, depending on what they think other athletes will do. The decision as to whether or not to use drugs might thus appear to be a problem for the individual athlete, but it can be better understood if it is seen as a coordination problem among all the players.

The Norwegian philosopher of sport Gunnar Breivik has been a central figure in the application of a variety of socio-psychological game models to the understanding of drug use in sport. These theoretical models of the 'doping game' (Breivik 1992: 235) regard drug use in sport as a 'decision dilemma', similar to the widely used 'prisoners' dilemma', and more particularly as a *moral* dilemma, for athletes who may have different values and preferences regarding the use of drugs, but who are thought to think and act rationally in order to maximize the likelihood of achieving what they regard as the best outcome for themselves when faced with the decision of whether or not to use drugs. This 'best outcome', it should be noted, will vary from one athlete to another, for while one athlete may define his/her best outcome in terms of winning the race, another athlete may define the best outcome simply in terms of competing 'clean' (Breivik 1992). A central underlying assumption of the game theoretical approach is that the use of performance-enhancing drugs is to a large extent an athlete-led and athlete-centred activity which results from the conscious (and morally based) decisions made by individual athletes within drug-using situations.

Breivik sets out the simplest model of a two-person doping dilemma as follows:

> Suppose doping is a ... game played ... between two of the best discus throwers in the world. Suppose they are Lombardian players who, like the famous American coach Vince Lombardi, believe that winning is the only thing that matters. Suppose that doping is efficient and increases the chances of winning. The best situation for a Lombardian player is that s/he dopes but the opponent does not dope. The second best is no-doping for both (since doping incurs costs). Next worst is doping for both. And worst is a situation where the opponent dopes but the Lombardian player does not dope.

He notes that the doping game with two Lombardian players would lead to doping as the dominant strategy. He adds:

> Since we know there are Lombardians in elite sport this preference ranking is crucial if one wants to understand and explain the use of doping. It also means that in order to combat doping one needs to change the preference rankings of Lombardians by increasing the risk and the costs of being caught and by increasing the benefits of playing fair.
>
> (Breivik 2015)

In Breivik's first (1987) paper, he examined different types of two-person games, but in a later paper (1992) he extended the analysis to n-person games. Later papers by Tangen and Breivik (2001), Haugen (2004), Kräkel (2007) and Eber (2008) have also developed more complex n-person game models which, it might be argued, more effectively take into account than did the earlier models the ways in which athletes' decision-making may be influenced by the wider structures of sport, such as the structure of financial and other rewards for winning and the system of detection and punishment.

Sporting careers, biographical risks and drug use

The German sociologist of sport Karl-Heinrich Bette has sought to offer a framework for understanding drug use in sport which centres on the issues of risk and risk reduction in athletic careers. Bette notes that our lives necessarily involve risks, since there is no life that can be fully planned and guided. However, he suggests that, in addition to the normal risks with which we all have to cope, athletes are also 'subject to special circumstances that appear neither in other social sectors nor, to a comparable degree, in the elite sport of an earlier period' (Bette 2004: 101). Bette goes on to identify what he calls the 'typical risk factors of athletic careers' and suggests that drug use can be seen as a 'coping strategy' that grows out of these specific risks.

Bette suggests that the increased risk factors in athletic careers are linked to the changed significance of contemporary sport. More particularly, he suggests that elite sport has become increasingly attractive to corporate interests, politicians and the mass media, and that this has been associated with 'the emergence of a constant demand for high-level sports performances, with the result that the role of risk-taking in athletic careers has taken on an entirely new role' (Bette 2004: 101). The major risk that is run by elite athletes is that they will not be successful in their careers. Although, as Bette notes, this statement at first sounds banal, it is important to note that a distinctive feature of athletic careers, and one which is found much less frequently in other careers, is that sporting competitions produce losers in a systematic way; indeed, athletic competition 'requires lots of losers so that the winners can distinguish themselves' (p. 102). And as global competition makes the intensity of competition increasingly fierce, so the risks of failure increase. In this regard, Bette (2004: 101) claims that 'the spread of doping is largely a consequence of the altered circumstances in which elite athletes pursue their careers', and of the ways and extent to which they continually attempt to manage the opportunities and risks that have become a part of their lives.

Risks in sport do not simply result from defeat in competition. Bette suggests that the 'high degree of uncertainty that characterizes athletic careers arises on account of something that distinguishes elite sport from other social enterprises in a very particular way, namely, the *extreme dependency on the body that marks the athletic enterprise*' (Bette 2004: 103; emphasis in the original). This means that an athlete has to establish an instrumental relationship to his/her body for, in the world of elite sport, 'career plans can be ruined overnight if the body refuses to perform' (p. 103). Every athlete thus runs the risk of failure on account of injuries, illness, declining performance or psychological 'burnout'.

Within this context, Bette suggests that in the modern sporting world, where the pursuit of enhanced sporting excellence at the elite level through the use of legitimate techniques such as specialized training and tactics has become increasingly limited, the growing prevalence of drug use is best seen 'not as an accidental aggregation of individual acts, but rather as a coping strategy which many athletes use in an attempt to counteract the risks they run' (Bette 2004: 107). Drug use in elite sport is thus seen to serve as '*a kind of multi-purpose weapon to prevent failure and to minimize the uncertainty about the future that comes in the wake of an athletic career*' (Bette 2004: 107; emphasis in the original). For a growing number of athletes, Bette suggests, the use of performance-enhancing drugs has become 'the procedure of choice' for managing the demands of elite sport, and particularly as a vehicle for eliminating 'the adverse effects of anxiety or excitement, to solve motivation problems, or to produce calm or relaxation in competitive situations' (Bette 2004: 107).

In addition to the perceived performance-related benefits the use of illicit drugs has for athletes, Bette contends, is the advantage it may give them within the struggle for scarce opportunities to obtain support, and particularly financial support, for both training and competing in their respective disciplines. Indeed, given the growing importance which athletes and clubs now attach to high-profile sporting competitions and the rewards with which they are so often associated, regular participation in such competitions is 'an indispensable prerequisite for staying at the elite level' (Bette 2004: 107). Thus, insofar as failure in high-level competitions 'involves the risk of not having access to these resources or of being cut off from them altogether' (Bette 2004: 107), athletes are said to be faced with the choice of deciding whether 'the risk of losing resources is greater or smaller than the risk of being caught' using performance-enhancing drugs (Bette 2004: 107). Bette also suggests that drug use by athletes can be seen as a strategy for managing and asserting their personal self-images and identities. In this regard, it is claimed that the 'performance-oriented individualism of today's individual elite athlete' (Bette 2004: 108) means that athletes are becoming increasingly constrained to portray positive self-images of themselves to others through being successful in their respective sports. The related pressures on athletes to be successful competitively and to meet the high expectations of coaches, sponsors and others (particularly in relation to the investment of substantial financial subsidies), is also cited as a reason why some athletes may seek, by using illicit drugs, to minimize the economic risks and uncertainties associated with what can, for many of them, be short careers. In this context, Bette suggests that, given the emphasis that has come to be placed upon winning in modern global sport, the increasing use of performance-enhancing drugs in elite sport is not surprising. In particular, he suggests that:

> lack of success presents a threat, not just to the individual athlete, but to everyone involved in producing performances. Coaches, officials, clubs and federations, corporate and political sponsors all have a stake in success. It is precisely those people who are professionally employed in elite sport and have no career alternatives who are under pressure to make sure that the athlete they either take care of or sponsor is successful no matter what. The coach's position and career are on the line; sports physicians are judged, not on whether they promote health, but on whether they have the athlete ready for competitions. For clubs and federations, state funding, payments from sponsors and perhaps television revenues are all at stake. And the sponsors need a continuous series of successes, because otherwise the public and potential advertisers will lose interest.
>
> (Bette 2004: 105)

Medical sociological approaches to drug use in sport

In the early 1990s, several authors began to draw attention to the importance of understanding the increasingly close relationship between medicine and sport as a basis for understanding drug use in sport. In his *Mortal Engines*, Hoberman (1992) argued that in the early years of the twentieth century, 'sport served the ends of science rather than the other way round', for sport was seen as just another form of human activity the study of which could aid our understanding of human physiology. In contrast to that earlier period, however, 'the modern outlook sees symbolic importance in the pursuit of the record performance, thereby putting physiology in the service of sport' (Hoberman 1992: 140). This was a critically important insight.

In the same year, Waddington and Murphy (1992) drew attention to the medicalization of the wider society as the essential context for understanding drug use, and also sought to analyse how, with the development of sports medicine, the medicalization process had encompassed sport itself. The following year, Lüschen (1993) also pointed to the medicalization of society in general as a contextual condition that 'sets the stage for legitimising the use of drugs in sport' (Lüschen 1993: 93). Waddington (1996) later extended the analysis of the development of sports medicine and its relationship to the development and use of performance-enhancing drugs in sport and since then Hoberman (2002, 2012, 2013) and Waddington (2000, 2001, 2004, 2005a, 2007; Waddington and Smith 2009), in a series of publications, have consistently drawn attention to the central role of sports physicians in the doping process. The central thrust of this approach thus focuses on developments in, and changes in the interrelationships between, medicine and sport and, more particularly, on changes in the relationship between sports physicians and athletes. A key element in this was the medicalization process.

The medicalization of life

In a classic essay of medical sociology, Irving Zola (1972) argued that in modern societies medicine is becoming a major institution of social control. This process, he argued, has been associated with the 'medicalizing' of much of daily living, a process which involves 'making medicine and the labels "healthy" and "ill" *relevant* to an ever increasing part of human existence' (Zola 1972: 487).

The theme of the medicalization of life was subsequently taken up by a number of other writers. Most notably, Ivan Illich argued that the medicalization of life involves a growing dependence on professionally provided care, growing dependence on drugs, medicalization of the life-span, medicalization of prevention and medicalization of the expectations of lay people. One of the consequences has been the creation of 'patient majorities' for, argued Illich (1975: 56), people 'who are free of therapy-oriented labels have become the exception'. Large numbers of people are now regarded as requiring routine medical attention, not because they have any definable pathology, but 'for the simple fact that they are unborn, newborn, infants, in their climacteric, or old' (Illich 1975: 44).

The medicalization of sport

In the last five decades or so – that is, very roughly, the period coinciding with the most rapid growth in the illicit use of drugs – the medicalization process has encompassed sport. This process has been most evident in the rapid development, particularly since the early 1960s, of sports medicine.

The medicalization of sport is clearly expressed in one of the first British texts in sports medicine, J.G.P. Williams's *Sports Medicine* (1962), in which the author asserts that the trained athlete 'is as different physiologically and psychologically from "the man in the street" as is the chronic invalid' and that '(j)ust as extreme youth and senility produce peculiar medical problems, so too does extreme physical fitness' (Williams 1962: vii). One can see here the early development of the idea, now widely accepted, that athletes require routine medical supervision not because they have any clearly defined pathology but, in this case, simply because they are athletes. Athletes thus became yet one more group to add to Illich's list of those – the unborn, newborn, infants and so on – who are held *by definition* to require routine medical supervision, irrespective of the presence or absence of any specific pathology.

One consequence of the development of the discipline of sports medicine, and of closely associated disciplines such as exercise physiology, biomechanics and sports psychology, has been to make top-class athletes more and more dependent on increasingly sophisticated systems of medical support in their efforts to run faster, to jump further or to compete more effectively in their chosen sport; indeed, at the highest levels, the quality of medical support may make the difference between success and failure. And, most importantly, this dependence of athletes on practitioners of sports medicine goes beyond the treatment of sports injuries for, as the British Medical Association's definition of sports medicine explicitly recognizes, sports medicine is concerned not just with the 'prevention, diagnosis, and treatment of exercise related illnesses and injuries' but also with the 'maximization of performance' (BMA 1996: 4). As Safai (2007: 326), writing about the development of sports medicine in Canada, has noted, sports medicine is now 'a tool to be used in the enhancement of athletes' performance in training and competition'.

Athletes are, however, not simply unwilling 'victims' of medical imperialism for, as de Swaan (1988: 246) has noted, professionals – in this instance, doctors – 'do not simply force themselves upon innocent and unknowing clients'. In the case of sport, a number of developments, particularly in the post-Second World War period, have led athletes increasingly to turn for help to anyone who can hold out the promise of improving their level of performance. The most important of these developments are those which have been associated with the commercialization of sport and the politicization of sport, both of which have been associated with massive increases in the rewards – particularly the material rewards – associated with sporting success. Both these processes have had the consequence of greatly increasing the value attached to winning.

In their history of sports in America since 1945 – significantly entitled *Winning is the Only Thing* – Roberts and Olsen (1989: xi–xii) note that, after 1945, Americans 'came to take sports very seriously, and they watched and played for the highest economic, politic, and personal stakes'. Similar changes have occurred elsewhere. In almost all countries, sport is now more competitive and more serious than it used to be, with a greater stress upon the importance of winning. Sport is played for higher – sometimes much higher – stakes, whether these be economic, political–national, personal or a combination of all three. This is an important part of the context for understanding the increasing cooperation between athletes and sports physicians in the search for medal-winning and record-breaking performances; as Houlihan (2002: 102) has noted, the development of sports medicine, 'coupled with the increasing pressures, from governments and commerce, on athletes to succeed has ... led to a deepening relationship between the athletes and the doctor … and, for most athletes, a growing dependence'.

The sport/medicine axis

This approach thus suggests that what is generally agreed to have been a significant increase in the illicit use of drugs since the 1960s (Miller 1996; Lüschen 2000; Donati 2004; Verroken 2005; Waddington and Smith 2009) has been associated with two key processes: (1) the 'medicalization of sport' and (2) the growing emphasis on the importance of winning. More specifically, developments within the medical profession have meant that medical practitioners have been increasingly prepared to make their professional knowledge and skills available to athletes at the very time when athletes, as a result of other developments within sport, have been increasingly eager to seek the help of scientists who can improve the level of their performance. The conjuncture of these two processes has been associated with two closely related developments. One of these developments – which is generally viewed as wholly legitimate – involves the emergence of sports medicine; the other – which is normally regarded as illegitimate – involves the increasing use by athletes of banned substances to improve their performance. The close association between these two developments had already been noted by Brown and Benner little more than 20 years after the publication of the first British textbooks in sports medicine. They noted that, as increased importance has been placed on winning, so athletes:

> have turned to mechanical (exercise, massage), nutritional (vitamins, minerals), psychological (discipline, transcendental meditation), and pharmacological (medicines, drugs) methods to increase their advantage over opponents in competition. A major emphasis has been placed on the non-medical use of drugs, particularly anabolic steroids, central nervous system stimulants, depressants and analgesics.
>
> (Brown and Benner 1984: 32)

It should be noted that since this approach stresses the conjuncture of two processes, one within the world of medicine and the other within the world of sport, it follows that the increasing use of drugs in sport *cannot be explained simply by reference to the changing patterns of behaviour among athletes*. Rather, this approach directs our attention to the development of a network of cooperative relationships between athletes who have been prepared to make illicit use of the fruits of medical and pharmacological research and sports physicians who have been prepared to stretch the boundaries of 'sports medicine' to include the prescribing of drugs with the specific intention of improving athletic performance. There is abundant evidence of the development of this network of cooperative relationships between the two increasingly closely related fields of sport and medicine.

Doctors as providers of 'chemical assistance': a brief history

Sports medicine is a legitimate area of specialist practice. There is, however, a substantial and well-documented body of evidence which confirms that 'physicians have played a significant, and largely unacknowledged, role in the doping of many elite athletes over the past 50 years' (Hoberman 2002: 203). It is not possible within the confines of this chapter to trace in detail the close relationship between the development of sports medicine and the development and use of performance-enhancing drugs (for more detail see Waddington 1996; Waddington and Smith 2009: 64–101; and Hoberman 2002, 2012) but what is clear is that, as Hoberman (2002: 207) has noted, 'the doping of athletes by sports physicians is more than a fringe phenomenon'. Well-documented early examples of the involvement of sports physicians in the development and use of performance-enhancing drugs are the central role of Dr John Ziegler, the US team doctor at the 1956 World Games in Moscow, in the development and dissemination among the weightlifting community of the first widely used anabolic steroids; the systematic involvement of doctors in doping in the former East Germany; and the involvement of sports medicine specialists in the development of blood doping (Waddington 1996). Hoberman (2012: 251–255) has also documented the emergence of a steroid lobby among sports physicians in West Germany during the 1980s.

As long ago as 1988, a leading UK medical journal, *The Lancet*, published an article under the title 'Sports medicine – is there lack of control?' It suggested that although 'evidence of direct involvement of medical practitioners in the procurement and administration of hormones is lacking, their connivance with those who do so is obvious and their participation in blood doping is a matter of record' (*Lancet* 1988: 612). We did not have to wait long for an abundance of evidence of the direct involvement of physicians in supplying drugs to athletes, for the Dubin Commission of Inquiry, established by the Canadian Government following Ben Johnson's infamous positive test at the 1988 Seoul Olympics, provided a detailed picture of the network of relationships between doctors, athletes and coaches in relation to drug use. Dubin (1990: 385) concluded that 'Physicians have played an important role in supplying anabolic steroids and other banned drugs to athletes. Many athletes who testified at this Inquiry received banned substances from physicians.' Hoberman (2012: 250) has correctly noted that this scenario 'has been confirmed over and over again in the course of the two decades that have elapsed since the Dubin Commission substituted documentation for speculation regarding doctors' direct involvement in the doping subculture'.

As Hoberman noted, the revelations in the Dubin report did little to disrupt what was by then a long-established pattern of cooperation between doctors and drug-using athletes. Eight years after the Dubin report was published, the drugs scandal in the 1998 Tour de France made it unambiguously clear that, once again, physicians – this time in the form of team doctors – were heavily implicated in the organization of drug use (Waddington 2000; Waddington and Smith

2009). Team doctors have also been implicated in the systematic use of drugs within professional football in Europe (Malcolm and Waddington 2008). As the British Medical Association (BMA) – not a body given to sensationalist statements – has noted, 'it is clear that, at the elite level, the involvement of team doctors in doping is not uncommon and that it has not been confined to the former communist countries of eastern Europe' (BMA, 2002: 84).

In recent years, the leading anti-doping campaigner Allessandro Donati has revealed details of the involvement of doctors in doping in Italian sport (Donati, 2004, 2006), while in 2006 the Spanish police uncovered an extensive blood-doping network which centred on the Madrid clinic of Dr Eufemiano Fuentes, who had been involved in blood doping perhaps as many as 200 elite athletes, including many of the world's leading cyclists (Waddington and Smith 2009: 81; Hoberman 2012: 256–257). In 2007 a major investigation into drug use in American baseball revealed that physicians were centrally involved in writing prescriptions for performance-enhancing drugs (Mitchell 2007). And in his autobiography, Tyler Hamilton, a former team mate of Lance Armstrong, confirmed yet again the central role of team doctors in doping in cycling (Hamilton and Coyle 2012). Indeed, there has hardly been a major drugs scandal in modern sport in which physicians have not been centrally involved.

Conclusion

As we noted at the outset, the several approaches outlined above are not mutually exclusive and many share overlapping or similar ideas about how we can best understand drug use in sport. For example, the starting point for all these approaches is that we can best understand the behaviour of drug-using athletes not by focusing on the athlete as an isolated individual, but by locating athletes within the network of relationships in which they are involved within sport. This means that, for example, a central thrust of the theory of differential association – the need to understand the subculture of drug-using athletes – is also integral to the other approaches. Similarly, all the approaches would accept that changes in the structure of modern sport – specifically the commercialization, commodification and politicization of sport, which have had the effect of increasing the competitiveness of modern sport and the emphasis which has come to be placed on winning – provide an essential context for understanding drug use in sport. While this is clearly the case for the Marxist, the deviant overconformity, the biographical risk and the medical sociological approaches, it is also the case that the more recent game models, while retaining a focus on the more-or-less rational decision-making process by athletes as to whether or not to use drugs, have also increasingly taken into account these broader social processes.

But of course there are also differences between these approaches. The game models focus, in a way in which the other approaches do not, on individual decision-making by athletes. The 'deviant overconformity' approach suggests that athletes who use drugs do not do so because they reject sporting values but, on the contrary, because of their 'deviant overconformity' to key aspects of the sport ethic, most notably the value attached to winning. Bette's biographical risks approach focuses on the way in which drug use may be understood as a way of reducing the high level of risk which is an intrinsic part of athletic careers. The medical sociological approach suggests that if we wish to understand drug use in sport then it is essential that we understand the centrality of the relationship between elite-level athletes and practitioners of sports medicine. However, acceptance of any one of these approaches does not necessarily imply a rejection of the others and we may well conclude that they all have a contribution to make to our understanding of drug use in sport.

References

Bette, K.-H. (2004) 'Biographical risks and doping', in J. Hoberman and V. Möller (eds) *Doping and Public Policy*, Odense, University of Southern Denmark, 101–111.

Breivik, G. (1987) 'The doping dilemma. Some game theoretical and philosophical considerations', *Sportwissenschaft*, 17, 83–94.

Breivik, G. (1992) 'Doping games. A game theoretical exploration of doping', *International Review for the Sociology of Sport*, 27, 235–256.

Breivik, G. (2015) 'Game theoretic approaches to doping in sport', in V. Möller, I. Waddington and J. Hoberman (eds) *Routledge Handbook of Drugs in Sport*, London, Routledge, 393–404.

BMA (British Medical Association), Board of Science and Education (1996) *Sport and Exercise Medicine: Policy and Provision*, London, British Medical Association.

BMA (British Medical Association) (2002) *Drugs in Sport: The Pressure to Perform*, London, British Medical Association.

Brohm, J.-M. (1978) *Sport – A Prison of Measured Time*, London, Ink Links.

Brown, T.C. and Benner, C. (1984) 'The nonmedical use of drugs', in W.N. Scott, B. Nisonson and J.A. Nicholas (eds) *Principles of Sports Medicine*, Baltimore and London, Williams & Wilkins.

Bryson, L. (1990), 'Sport, drugs and the development of modern capitalism', *Sporting Traditions*, 6, 135–153.

Coakley, J. (2007) *Sports in Society: Issues and Controversies*, ninth edition, New York, McGraw-Hill.

de Swaan, A. (1988) *In Care of the State*, Cambridge, Cambridge University Press.

Donati, A. (2004) 'The silent drama of the diffusion of doping among amateurs and professionals', in J. Hoberman and V. Møller (eds), *Doping and Public Policy*, Odense, University Press of Southern Denmark, 45–90.

Donati, A. (2006). 'Doping and doping control in Italian sport', in G. Spitzer (ed.) *Doping and Doping Control in Europe*, Oxford, Meyer and Meyer, 17–56.

Dubin, The Hon. Charles L. (1990) *Commission of Inquiry into the Use of Drugs and Banned Practices Intended to Increase Athletic Performance*, Ottawa, Canadian Government Publishing Centre.

Eber, N. (2008) 'The performance-enhancing drug game reconsidered. A fair play approach', *Journal of Sports Economics*, 9, 318–327.

Hamilton, T. and Coyle, D. (2012) *The Secret Race*, London, Bantam Press.

Haugen, K.K. (2004) 'The performance-enhancing drug game', *Journal of Sports Economics*, 5, 67–86.

Hoberman, J. (1992) *Mortal Engines*, New York, Free Press.

Hoberman, J. (2002) 'Sports physicians and the doping crisis in elite sport', *Clinical Journal of Sport Medicine*, 12, 203–208.

Hoberman, J. (2003) ' "A pharmacy on wheels": doping and community cohesion among professional cyclists following the Tour de France scandal of 1998', in V. Møller and J. Nauright (eds) *The Essence of Sport*, Odense, University Press of Southern Denmark, 107–127.

Hoberman, J. (2012) 'Sports physicians and doping: medical ethics and elite performance', in D. Malcolm and P. Safai, *The Social Organization of Sports Medicine*, New York, Routledge, 237–264.

Hoberman, J. (2013) 'Sports physicians, human nature, and the limits of medical enhancement', in J. Tolleneer, S. Sterckx and P. Bonte (eds) *Athletic Enhancement, Human Nature and Ethics*, Dordrecht, Springer, 255–270.

Houlihan, B. (2002) *Dying to Win: Doping in Sport and the Development of Anti-doping Policy*, second edition, Strasbourg, Council of Europe.

Illich, I. (1975) *Medical Nemesis*, London, Calder & Boyars.

Kräkel, M. (2007) 'Doping and cheating in contest-like situations', *European Journal of Political Economy*, 23, 988–1006.

Lancet (1988) 'Sports medicine – is there lack of control?', *The Lancet*, 2, 612.

Lüschen, G. (1993) 'Doping in sport: the social structure of a deviant subculture', *Sport Science Review*, 2 (1), 92–106.

Lüschen, G. (2000) 'Doping in sport as deviant behaviour and its social control', in J. Coakley and E. Dunning (eds) *Handbook of Sports Studies*, London, Sage, 461–476.

Malcolm, D. and Waddington, I. (2008) ' "No systematic doping in football"; a critical review', *Soccer in Society*, 9 (1), 198–214.

Miller, A.P. (1996) 'Drugs in sport', *Journal of Performance Enhancing Drugs*, 1 (3), 106–112.

Mitchell, G. (2007) *Report to the Commissioner of Baseball of an Independent Investigation into the Illegal Use of Steroids and other Performance Enhancing Substances by Players in Major League Baseball*, New York, Office of the Commissioner of Baseball.

Monaghan, L. F. (2001) *Bodybuilding, Drugs and Risk*, London, Routledge.

Nixon, H.L. II (1992) 'A social network analysis of influences on athletes to play with pain and injuries', *Journal of Sport and Social Issues*, 16 (2), 127–135.

PMP Consultancy (2001) *Studies to Combat Doping in Sport*, Lot 3, Final Report, Brussels, European Commission.

Rigauer, B. (1981) *Sport and Work*, New York, Columbia University Press.

Roberts, R. and Olsen, J. (1989) *Winning is the Only Thing*, Baltimore, Johns Hopkins University Press.

Safai, P. (2007) 'A critical analysis of the development of sport medicine in Canada, 1955–80', *International Review for the Sociology of Sport*, 42, 321–341.

Sutherland, E. and Cressey, D. (1974) *Criminology*, Philadelphia, Lippincott.

Tangen, J.O. and Breivik, G. (2001) 'Doping games and drug abuse. A study of the relation between preferences, strategies, and behavior in relation to doping in Norwegian sports', *Sportwissenschaft*, 31, 188–198.

Verroken, M. (2005) 'Drug use and abuse in sport', in D. Mottram (ed.) *Drugs in Sport*, fourth edition, London, Routledge.

Waddington, I. (1996) 'The development of sports medicine', *Sociology of Sport Journal*, 13 (2), 176–196.

Waddington, I. (2000) *Sport, Health and Drugs*, London and New York, E. & F.N. Spon.

Waddington, I. (2001) 'Doping in sport: a medical sociological perspective', in Research Council of Norway, *Research on Doping in Sport*, Oslo, Research Council of Norway, 11–21.

Waddington, I. (2004) 'Doping in sport: some issues for medical practitioners', in J. Hoberman and V. Møller (eds) *Doping and Public Policy*, Odense, University Press of Southern Denmark, 31–44.

Waddington, I. (2005a) 'Le dopage sportif: la responsibilité des praticiens médicaux', *Revue internationale des sciences du sport et de l'education*, 9–23.

Waddington, I. (2005b) 'Changing patterns of drug use in British sport from the 1960s', *Sport in History*, 25 (3), 472–496.

Waddington, I. (2007) 'Doping in de sport – naar een sociologische verklaring', in J. Van Gestel (ed.) *Figuraties in de sport*, Gent, Academia Press, 185–211.

Waddington, I. and Murphy, P. (1992) 'Drugs, sport and Ideologies', in E. Dunning and C. Rojek (eds) *Sport and Leisure in the Civilizing Process*, Basingstoke, Macmillan, 36–64.

Waddington, I. and Smith, A. (2009) *An Introduction to Drugs in Sport: Addicted to Winning?* London, Routledge.

Williams, J. (1962) *Sports Medicine*, London, Edward Arnold.

Zola, I. (1972) 'Medicine as an institution of social control', *Sociological Review*, n.s. 20, 487–504.

3 "The winner takes it all" – individualization and performance and image enhancing in sport and in society

Nader Ahmadi and Göran Svedsäter

Background

News media give us independent evidence of the existence of sports doping. The problems are widespread and likely growing. Within the world of sports and physical culture, these trends are rather easy to observe. The fixation with one's own body, and the conceptions about what is the ideal body on the one hand, and the immense economic benefits of being top in sports on the other, might be among the contributing factors to young people's justifying the use of doubtful and even illegal means of reaching the ideals of success and beauty. The article illustrates doping in society, specifically doping outside sports, with the focus on use of performance-and image-enhancing drugs/substance (PIED), especially anabolic androgenic steroids (AAS).

It appears that the use of PIED occurs not only in sport but also in the wider community. The misuse of doping substances in wider society has to be clearly differentiated from doping in elite sport and, to some degree, also from doping in recreational sport, as their motives differ (Mickelsson, 2009). The ideals of health and fitness in today's society have to be understood and dissected, since these ideals, paradoxically, could lead to increased use of doping substances in the quest for better physical performance, appearance and/or self-esteem.

Individualism characterizes the Western style of life, and emanates from the individual and his or her needs, something that stands in contrast to collectivism, which instead emphasizes the group's objectives as the most important (Frisén *et al.*, 2014).

Being part of a culture that emphasizes individualism influences the individual's view of his or her own body. In an individualistic culture which is often marked by affluence, it is important to have personal self-realization, where the body and appearance are important components.

Thereby a social pressure builds up on individuals to take care of their own bodies, where appearance and matching the beauty ideal is a symbol of success (Frisén *et al.*, 2014).

In this context, food supplements, the slimming culture, beauty surgery, etc., can be regarded as methods in a society where increased individualization has entailed that change and manipulation of body/appearance to achieve the ideal/perfection has become existential.

Generation performance

Within sport, the use of doping has been motivated by the fact that the athlete wishes to improve his or her performance and thereby achieve better results than the individual's normal ability would indicate.

However, in today's society there is the "phenomenon" that contributes to a sharper focus on "the perfect life." An increased individualization results in an increased body focus and obsession with bodily and appearance perfectionism. Competition and elitism are associated with this context and influence the ideal that many young people are trying to achieve; self-image, body image, beauty ideals and masculinity ideals are central components. Such "winning culture" influences the individual to use doping and other available means in order to achieve success as quickly as possible.

Use of illegal substances such as AAS to improve performance is not a new phenomenon; on the contrary, it can be established that non-medical use of AAS, which previously largely took place within sport, has moved out to other target groups in society that are not primarily motivated by sports-related performance (Sagoe *et al.*, 2015).

Doping outside sport is thereby no longer only a medical misuse problem, but also a symbol of a society where the emphasis is on changing/manipulating the body so that the individual's appearance matches a type of ideal, as well as improving physical performance.

In our society it is emphasized that the individual should be competent, function well socially, and have a beautiful body and appearance. This applies especially to the younger generation, who experience a society with increased body pressure. There is an especially extensive focus on the body and appearance, and the media, as well as advertising, play a decisive role by accentuating ideal bodies, meaning that many young people do a lot to achieve this ideal. For generating performance, training at a "fitness center" is closely connected to performance of the body, and a wish to perform in all areas of life. Training and being a part of the fitness culture of our time has become an important part of personal image, communicated by social media, motivation and not only training, but also talking about it. Being healthy with a well-trained and muscular body has become an important factor in our society, indicating that the individual is successful and has a large amount of self-confidence (Youth Support Team, 2015).

Individuals who feel that their body and appearance do not match the beauty ideal that is presented by society in different ways can come to use performance-enhancing drugs or methods to improve their appearance, especially to become more muscular. In this way, having complexes about the appearance or size of the body can be a motivation to start doping (Barland and Tangen, 2009).

With such a starting point it will probably be a connection between how the body is perceived and the use of muscle-building substances (Singhammer and Ibsen, 2010).

The longing for "perpetual youth" leads to a society where finding the source of youth takes new forms. A new contribution to this is the increase in sales of testosterone supplements. The target group is middle-aged men, and use aims to counteract a natural ageing process and entail a form of "perpetual youth." Testosterone sales have increased substantially, particularly among older men, during recent years (Handelsman, 2012).

Occurrence of doping in society

Explanations of why active and health-conscious individuals are willing to take the risks entailed by using preparations such as AAS are complex.

Users outside sports are mainly divided into three groups – athletes, estheticians and perpetrators of crimes. But there are also other reasons for using doping preparations. The majority of those who use AAS are men between the ages of 18 and 34 and usage is much lower among women (Mickelsson, 2009).

> The principal purpose of athletes who use dope has always been to increase athletic performance through better strength, power, speed, increased muscle size and explosivity. Perpetrators of crimes use AAS to achieve a greater body volume, increased strength and often aggressiveness, which entail better possibilities to fight as well as frighten. On the other hand, estheticians use AAS primarily to improve their appearance, become strong and achieve the beauty ideal to which they aspire.
>
> (Mickelsson, 2009, p.12)

It is not clear how widespread the use of doping preparations is. Data from Customs and the Police shows the number of confiscations, illegal importation and illegal sales indicate that the phenomenon is far more usual and more extensive than the number of users discovered by the surveys (Mickelsson, 2009; Hoff, 2013).

It can be seen from a recently published Norwegian study that an average of 2.1 percent of the Nordic population have used anabolic steroids (AAS) at least once (Sagoe *et al.*, 2015). In addition, an international study show that 3.3 percent of the world's population has used AAS at least once (Sagoe *et al.*, 2014).

The discrepancy that exists between the proven number of users and confiscation/sales, as well as information from other institutions, indicates that use of doping preparations outside sport is more extensive than has been assumed.

Therefore, use of doping outside sport has received greater attention in the last few years.

Individualism and individualization

The rise of the individual as the core of society and the individualization of different spheres of human society is regarded as one of the consequences of modernity (Giddens, 1990; Bauman, 1998, 2001; Beck and Beck-Gernsheim, 2012; Dumont, 1992). Modern sociological classics normally view individualism as predominantly positive. Individualism is perceived as a way of understanding the self and the self's relationships to the other as democratic, freed from hierarchy and enhancing individuals' opportunities to realize themselves/possibilities/abilities. General humanity as the point of departure was replaced by the individual. Individualism is built on the idea of individuals as independent, self-sufficient, rational, autonomous entities with certain economic, political and legal rights, who together with other individuals with the same rights and obligations constitute a society. The individual, here, is conceived in terms of a "place in a system of social relations" and society is considered in terms of a compound of "individualist individuals," or the individuals who have internalized a certain concept of person, a concept according to which each individual is in the last instance more important than any larger constituent group (Dumont, 1992; Mauss, 1985; Ahmadi and Ahmadi, 1998). Even in the dawn of modernity, Weber identified rationalism as an inherent characteristic of modernity.

Although we have witnessed several historical processes of modernization, leading to different forms and levels of modernity, we might maintain that during the last four decades, many societies, both Western and non-Western, have been characterized by what many refer to as a second modernity (Beck, 1992) or late modernity (Giddens, 1991) or post-modernity (Lyotard, 1993). Whatever name is used, one can distinguish an intensified individualization, an increased instrumentalization of interpersonal relationships and a radical shift of values towards an absolute dominance of market values (Swader, 2008) as the common characteristics of this level of modernity.

This intensified individualization is referred to as an extreme form of individualism focusing on the personal ambitions, will and motivations/derivations of individuals not in relation to a normative other-oriented context – an institutionalized individualism, as Bauman (2012) puts it (in Beck and Beck-Gernsheim, 2012), which focuses on strategies that increase chances for personal success/gain, self-reflexivity, with indifference towards others and normative regulations. A purely rational cost–benefit analysis is the basis of individualization. "The ideological notion of the self-sufficient individual ultimately implies the disappearance of any sense of mutual obligations" (p. xxi): a conflict of values, with the self as the supreme value object. Individualism regards the individual per se as the value object; however, the bottom-line value object for individualization is the self.

The market economy in its pure form induces profit-oriented thinking and self-centeredness leading to pragmatic rationality becoming liberated from its moral roots. As we mentioned earlier, economic cultures have a formative impact in relation to patterning values, ways of thinking and consequently personalities and life ideals. However, it does not stop there – different economic and cultural systems promote and sanction certain sets of action and ways of thinking – a cultural influence or imposition, so to speak.

In the context of today's economy and money culture, the self-oriented values encourage a rational and instrumental approach to means of reaching success. If modern society was the residue of the producers – a "producers' society" – and the late/second or post-modern society was conceived of as a society inhabited by consumers – a "consumers' society" (Bauman, 1998) – our contemporary society can be defined as the "winners' society." In a system of values where the valuation of winning is a rational and terminal concern, maximization of bodily performance within the athletic sphere can consequently be a means of achieving this end, although by means of doping. The goal justifies the means as long as one is not detected. The ethos of this society proclaims: if you win, you are pardoned. Winning is the path to salvation. In every aspect of modern life, from politics to sports, we witness this ethos. Political parties and politicians with dubious, dark pasts and ideologies become acceptable when they win. Winning-oriented pragmatic rationality, instrumentalization of interpersonal relations and exploitation of medical and scientific innovations, together with a culture of image-cultivation and consumerist display of luxuries, might explain the explosion of the use of illegal performance-enhancing methods in society in general and in sport in particular. Change of values and consequently individuals' way of thinking towards a more egocentric and rational pragmatic direction, combined with the commercialization of sport and the big money related to the elite athlete, paves the way for adaptation of instrumental values, focused on the means of attaining the particular end of winning at any price.

As the discussions above imply, the way individualization is referred to in this chapter (and by some other researchers, such as Beck and Beck-Gernsheim (2012), Bauman (2012) and Swader (2008)) is characterized not by an unreservedly positive view but as loaded with an essential criticism.

System of values and economic culture

It is commonly held that modernity has made people more self-centered, materialistic and rationalistic. Although it is difficult to empirically investigate a direct correlation between a society's prevailing ways of thinking and value systems on the one hand, and the current material and political movements in this society on the other, it is plausible to assume that economic, political and social systems influence the dominant values of society and the dominant ways of thinking of the people living in that society. In other words, just as value systems affect our economic and political behavior, the politics and economic culture of our time and our society, so they affect and shape our ways of thinking, value systems and behavior. One might say that economic systems promote not only their own behavioral patterns but also their specific cultural forms and ways of thinking.

Way of thinking, in general, comprises the ways in which people make value judgments and practical decisions, classify their experiences and establish relationships with their surroundings, etc. The phrase "way of thinking" refers to any individual's thinking in which the characteristic features of the thinking habits of the culture to which he or she belongs are revealed (Nakamura, 1971; Ahmadi and Ahmadi, 1998). In other words, the way of thinking is a magazine embracing the empirical aspects of the life of a people in a certain period of time.

Values are the basis for an individual's prioritizations for her/his actions. According to Swader, "values should be seen as the individual's prioritized internationalization of social norms used to guide his/her behavior" (2008, p. 33). Values emerge in the intersection between ways of thinking and sets of action/behavior. "[T]his value conception allows room for both agency and structure, as values are not merely handed down hierarchically, but are formed by individuals' perceptions of and reactions to concretized values within cultural systems" (p. 2). Values steer, to a large extent, our behaviors, choices, actions and priorities in our overall social interactions. Systems of values give rise to the tools that best serve them. A system of values, based on a pure market economy culture, of pursuing success, money and fame justifies tools necessary for achieving these goals. The valuation of reaching financial success/winning is a rational and terminal concern wherein maximization of chances to achieve the goals of success is the dominant form of behavior.

During recent decades society has undergone a rapid ideological and value change in the direction of enhanced individualization. It is therefore plausible to assume that the contemporary unchallenged victory of the market economy and the capitalist culture and value system[1] has contributed to a change in the society's value system toward a more individualized, instrumentalist system where individuals have become more self-oriented, materialistic and rationalistic. The individual's growing self-centeredness is articulated in her/his endeavor to maximize her/his self-gain through rational choices and by using rational calculation. The individual chooses what she/he understands as the most efficient means toward whatever end she/he is striving for with her/his specific actions. The market economy value system is manifested in a strong ethos of winning and/or success. In this value system, individuals' adaptation to the economy culture allows the domination of a culture of winning at any price. In other words, the market economy culture and ethos of success pattern the ways of thinking of individuals, who have already become self-oriented by the forces of modernity, toward an even more intensified self-centeredness.

It appears to be an imperative to act according to a kind of pragmatic rationality, otherwise the individual is regarded as irrational. And the morality of pragmatic rationality supports this way of thinking. It is an imperative to be successful, rich, and number one. Of course, the attractions of the luxurious life created by this success and the money related to it also constitute an additional weighty argument. Consequently, individuality becomes a burden when the expanded responsibility (read obligation) of the individual shapes his/her life.

The greater the responsibility, the greater the pressure and the greater his/her desperation to achieve success at any price, the more probable it is that the individual will use even legally prohibited means to achieve his/her goals. The norm our society holds up to its members is to be a winner. Present-day society loads its members with the duty to win, to be number one. To win is a must in this culture, yet the individual must reveal him/herself to that culture in the disguise of a freedom of will. The winner mentality and winner behavior become life's cognitive and moral centers, the ways in which people integrate into society and the main tools for controlling the system.

Personal success, economic and otherwise, has become in this system of values the ultimate value, replacing many societal moral values. Since wealth and success are considered as the ultimate values, this gives a de facto legitimation of the means of achieving them. Individuals are being socialized to the ethos of success and the means of achieving it: cost–benefit analysis, image cultivation, instrumentalization, celebrity pursuit. In this culture of success at any price, medical and technological developments open up new possibilities for enhancing performance in various areas of life. Not only athletes but many people in the general population use various pharmaceutical, medical and surgical, and technological/genetic technological means to increase physical as well as other types of performance in order to increase their chances of success (Breivik *et al.*, 2009). As Breivik *et al.* maintain,

> the ideas of natural body and natural ways to improve performance do not seem very widely held. A considerable number of people are willing to use enhancements and body modifications … the athletes and the population are more similar in their attitudes than one might expect.
>
> (p. 749)

These new possibilities can be related to an increasing demand, which in its turn is a result of value changes and self-centeredness. The developments within sport reflect the attitudes and practices of enhancement and body modification in wider society. In spite of bans and regulations, the use of drugs seems to be prevalent.

The media and the ethos of winning

The market culture, with its ethos of winning, consumerism and glorification of the luxurious life, creates its own conceptions of identity. If in pre-modern society it was the clan, the family and religion which were the determinants of people's identities, and if in the modern era profession and individual life-projects gave individuals their identity, in today's global society the quest for identity is through fame. A culture of winning forms the identity of the individual in the form of belonging to celebrity. Since the number of contenders bidding for a share of attention, a place in the sun, being someone, is growing at an exceptional pace in our global digital world, to be someone is to "win" an identity. Fame has replaced identity.

The media plays a crucial role in transferring market values and furthering individualization. The propaganda for the economy culture and market values has a manipulative effect on our ways of thinking. Different means of expression of popular culture (TV shows, movies, music and so on) sell ideals which are aligned with the culture of economic success and manipulate our values. Images of celebrity culture, showing the lifestyle and behavior of celebrities, invade our lives. Reality shows where any devaluation of values is accepted as long as it leads to economic benefits and celebrity (read success) for the participants prepare us for winning at any price. "Everything is forgiven if you achieve success" is the manifestation of a culture of amorality related to that success. It makes it easier to give up one's own moral scruples in the perspective of future fame, money and success. The use of performance-enhancing drugs in sport can be intimately linked to the value change and the dominating economic culture of society: "the use of banned drugs and methods can be considered a rational strategy" (Breivik *et al.*, 2009, p. 739). Those who choose to use illegal performance-enhancing drugs know that they are doing "wrong" but still *choose* to do it: the rationale is "if I don't get caught and still succeed, so much the better." According to a rational choice worldview (regardless of whether it concerns athletic activities or activities in society at large), the behavioral pattern is simply to find the most appropriate means to achieve the goals. Doping can be completely understood as a matter of rational calculation. On the other hand, society also tends to excuse those who win and are successful, rich and beautiful.

The fact that many athletes still adhere to the principles of anti-doping corresponds to the societal rules of the game by which individuals should adapt their behavior in certain ways in order to be successful within the capitalist economy. Profit-oriented pragmatic rationality, a high degree of personal ambition and independent self-sufficiency – each of these generates its own unique individualizing effect. The rational–pragmatic value system and the related way of thinking with its means-and-ends-focused forms of quantitative valuation are tools of success.

Increased individualization in society has entailed a larger focus on individuals' self-image, body perception and beauty ideal. The media, periodicals and commercial products both influence and strengthen a development where body and appearance has become something one should change. Such changing culture is in strong contrast to basic inter-human values such as tolerance and the belief that each person is unique in him- or herself.

> The media especially, but also other parts of society, place great emphasis on the body. The feminine and the masculine ideal are spread through advertising and other marketing. It is illegal to advertise doping, but it is possible to show photos of well-built, muscular bodies or to market food supplements with promises that one can achieve these ideals. The use of unnatural methods to improve appearance has become more usual and more accepted. That the social climate supports corrections of appearance also

contributes to use of doping substances. The ideal of beauty and health is also strengthened by society's performance culture.

(Mickelsson, 2009. p.26)

Conclusions

A common misconception in today's society is that everything is (or should be) rational and goal-oriented, which we summarized earlier as pragmatic rationalism. We call this pragmatic rationalism a misconception because it misses a historical fact that individuals' actions are and have never been governed entirely by rational motives. Emotional, ethical and existential considerations influence human actions extensively. Solidarity, willingness to share and even self-sacrifice and prioritizing the good of others before one's own are values that have survived many different economic cultures. Even today's extremely individualized society with its focus on reaching success and winning at any price cannot completely suppress these values. There is an inherent contradiction between the crude egoism of modern individualism and its historical development that largely has its origin in the care of humans. Although individualism is ultimately about respect for and protection of individuals' own prosperousness and interests, on a deeper level it is based on values other than purely selfish ones. Amarita Sen interprets this as the ethics-related view of motivation: "The first [issue] concerns the link between human motivation and the general ethical question how should one live?" (Sen, 1987, p. 28). To emphasize this relationship does not mean to claim that people always act in ways that they morally defend, but only to recognize that ethical considerations cannot be irrelevant for human behavior. This might contribute to building a broader view of the individual's best that does not only stem from the ethos of success materialized in the form of medals, money or glory.

Although individuals are believed to behave rationally, the question is what the content of the rational behavior is and who defines this content. It seems that the dominant tendency is to "identify rationality with maximization of self-interest" (Sen, 1987, p. 37). Trying one's best to achieve what one wants to achieve is regarded as the core of rationality. This means that egoistic behavior can be regarded as the sole basis for an economic, rational choice.

Is it by policing and police-inspired methods that WADA's anti-doping work should be carried out, or by changing the approach of the athletes from focusing on their own interests to the question "How should one live?"? The main question is: can doping can ever be stopped? Can this goal possibly be achieved in sport at all, if there is no parallel work at the community level at large taking a similar approach? Or will we find ourselves in an eternal struggle between the control bodies and the dopers?

Note

1 Of course, we are aware of the fact that there is no unitary market and economy culture. What we refer to here is an ideal type in the Weberian sense of the word. Furthermore, to avoid misunderstandings, we would like to make a clarification before we move on. We are not taking any standpoint against the development of individualism and modernity; on the contrary, we are convinced that modernity and individualism constitute an important historical development.

References

Ahmadi, N. and Ahmadi, F. (1998). *Iranian Islam: The Concept of the Individual*. Houndmills, Basingstoke: Macmillan.

Barland, B. and Tangen, J.O. (2009). *Kroppspresentasjon og andre prestasjoner- en omfangsundersøkelse om bruk av doping* (Presentation of the body and other performances: a national study on the use of drugs among youths). Oslo: Politihøgskolen Forskning, 3.2.

Bauman, Z. (1998). *Globalization: The Human Consequences*. Cambridge: Polity Press.

Bauman, Z. (2001). *The Individualized Society*. Cambridge: Polity Press.

Bauman, Z. (2012). Foreword: Individually, together, in U. Beck and E. Beck-Gernsheim, *Individualization*. London: Sage.

Beck, U. (1992). *Risk Society: Towards a New Modernity*. London: Sage.

Beck, U. and Beck-Gernsheim, E. (2012). *Individualization*. London: Sage.

Breivik, G., Hanstad, D.V. and Loland, S. (2009). Attitudes towards use of performance-enhancing substances and body modification techniques: a comparison between elite athletes and the general population. *Sport in Society*, 12 (6), 737–754.

Dumont, L. (1992). *Essays on Individualism*. Chicago: University of Chicago Press.

Frisén, A., Holmqvist Gattario, K. and Lunde, C. (2014). *Projekt perfekt. Om utseendekultur och kroppsuppfattning* (Project Perfect. Designating Culture and Body Image). Stockhjolm: Natur och Kultur.

Giddens, A. (1990). *The Consequences of Modernity*. Stanford: Stanford University Press.

Giddens, A. (1991). *Modernity and Self-Identity: Self and Society in the Late Modern Age*. Cambridge: Polity Press.

Handelsman, D. (2012). Pharmacoepidemiology of testosterone prescribing in Australia, 1992–2010. *Medical Journal of Australia* 196 (10), 642–645. doi: 10.5694/mja11.

Hoff, D. (2013). Doping outside sports – individualisation and muscular beauty ideals: a study of elementary schools, high schools and fitness centres in Kalmar municipality. *Scandinavian Sport Studies Forum*, 4, 1–24.

Lyotard, J.F. (1993). *The Postmodern Condition: A Report on Knowledge*. Minneapolis: University of Minnesota Press.

Mauss, M. (1985). A category of the human mind: the notion of person; the notion of self, in M. Carrithers, S. Collins and S. Lukes (eds) *The Category of Person: Anthropology, Philosophy, History*. Cambridge: Cambridge University Press.

Mickelsson, K. (2009). *Doping in Sweden: An Inventory of Spread, Consequences and Measures*. Rapport 2009:15. Östersund: Statens folkhälsoinstitut.

Nakamura, H. (1971). *Ways of Thinking of Eastern Peoples: India, China, Tibet, Japan*. Honolulu: University of Hawai'i Press.

Robins, K. and Webster, F. (1989). *The Technical Fix: Education, Computers and Industry.* London: Macmillan.

Sagoe, D., Torsheim, T., Molde, H., Andreassen, C.S. and Pallesen, S. (2015). Anabolic-androgenic steroid use in the Nordic countries: a meta-analysis and meta-regression analysis. *Nordic Studies on Alcohol and Drugs*, 32 (1). Early bird.

Sagoe, D., Molde, H., Andreassen, C. S., Torsheim, T., & Pallesen, S. (2014): The global epidemiology of anabolic-androgenic steroid use: A meta-analysis and meta-regression analysis. *Annals of Epidemiology*, 24, 383–398.

Sen, A. (1987). *On Ethics and Economics*. Oxford: Basil Blackwell.

Singhammer, J. and Ibsen, B., (2010). Motionsdoping i Danmark. En kvantitativ undersøgelse om brug af og holdning til muskelopbyggende stoffer (Exercise doping in Denmark. A quantitative study on the use of and attitude towards muscle-building substances). Center for forskning i Idræt, Sundhet og Civilsamfund, Syddansk Universitet.

Swader, C.S. (2008). Transformation to a market economy and changing social values in China, Russia, and Eastern Germany. Dissertation, University of Bremen.

Youth Support Team (2015). *Ungdom, Kropp og doping* (Youth, Kropp and Doping). Report 01/2015. Asker: Youth Support Team.

4 Reflections on 'doping in sport' and 'doping in society'

David Hoff

Introduction

Doping in sport is recognized as an important problem in relation to fair play and health. Anti-doping work in sport has been going on since the beginning of the 1960s, and has been accentuated on several occasions by 'doping scandals'. Until recently doping has been addressed solely as an internal sport issue, and not as a social problem outside sport. However, increasing evidence is showing that doping outside the elite sports context without any competitive reasons is not uncommon. Frequent use of anabolic androgenic steroids (AAS) has been reported at gyms, among high school and college students, in criminal contexts and in relation to other types of substance abuse – where the competitive reasons for using illicit performance enhancing substances are of minor importance. Instead, the use of doping substances such as AAS is motivated by cosmetic reasons (to be more muscular, gain or loss weight), by criminal strategic reasons (to be stronger and more fearsome) and as a component in general substance-abuse behaviour. The use of 'doping in society' has been acknowledged in research, but still the issue is not publicly well known, and anti-doping efforts, prevention programmes and treatment strategies are underdeveloped, contrary to what is going on in relation to doping in sport. There is a need for more research on how widespread doping is outside sport, on social driving forces and motives for use of different doping preparations, and on physiological, psychological and social consequences of its use.

In this article I discuss four issues in relation to the use of doping preparations – both within and outside sport (in society). In the first section – 'Different types of doping and reasons for doping' – I argue that 'doping in sport' differs from 'doping in society'. For instance, doping in sport is something different from doping in a criminal context. But there are also common dominators between different types of doping behaviours, which will be discussed in the article. In the second section – 'Doping use has to be understood in its own right' – I argue that there are specific elements in the doping behaviour that differentiate use of doping preparations from substance abuse (alcohol and narcotics). In the third section – 'Doping use is a sign of the times' – I am arguing that the use of doping preparations should not only be analysed from an individual perspective.

Until now, many studies have analysed doping as an individual problem (e.g. individual morals, a pessimistic personality, a risk-taking personality). I argue we have to consider the significance of current social processes and ideals in society to fully understand the interest in doping, not least concerning doping outside the competitive sports context. In the article I discuss some important social processes in relation to doping. In the fourth and last discussion I focus on today's strong health ideals in society, in the section 'The pursuit of good health could become unhealthy'. I argue that this is a double-edged development in relation to doping. To strive for better health through physical activities and a more healthy diet is of course a good thing, but when training and dieting become an obsession this can lead to eating disorders as well as use of doping substances.

Different types of doping and reasons for doping

There is not only one reason for using doping substances, there are several. Doping in elite sports has to be differentiated from doping in recreational sports, and doping in sport has to be differentiated from doping without any sporting ambitions, since the motives diverge. In elite sports the most common motives for use of doping preparations are to improve physical performance, to win competitions, for financial gain, to solve weight problems and to reduce pain (Backhouse *et al.*, 2007). In recreational sport at fitness centres and in gyms the most common motive for doping use is to build a more muscular and beautiful body (Backhouse *et al.*, 2007; Hoff, 2008). Outside sport, the use and abuse of performance enhancing drugs, especially AAS, has emerged as a social problem linked to substance abuse and crime (Mickelsson, 2009). Research studies have associated the use of AAS with aggression, violence and criminality where the motives have to do with strategic reasons: to be stronger and more fearsome (Johansson *et al.*, 2000; Lindqvist *et al.*, 2002; Mickelsson, 2009; Moberg and Hermansson, 2006; Skårberg, 2009; Thiblin and Pärlklo, 2002). Several studies have also suggested a connection between so-called risk behaviours, like abuse of alcohol and narcotics, and use of doping preparations (Kindlundh *et al.*, 1999; Papadopoulos *et al.*, 2006; Skårberg, 2009; Wichstrøm, 2006).

Owing to social problems with the use of doping, Sweden was the first nation in Europe to implement legislation concerning doping (Act 1991: 1969), which prohibits selling as well as using AAS and growth hormone (Mickelsson, 2009). The legislation is primarily directed towards doping behaviour outside the sports competition context. In sport, doping is regulated within the international sports community. Both seizures by Customs and prosecutions under the Act have increased several times since the implementation of the law (Hermansson and Moberg, 2008; Mickelsson, 2009). This increase in doping cases does not reflect the sport-specific doping control system, where only a few individuals are prosecuted every year in Sweden.

Studies of doping use outside competitive sport are few, and we still do not know much about the individuals and groups who are using doping substances.

We also lack knowledge on how widespread the use is, when it begins, and the motives of users. Nevertheless, studies which do exist have shown that a large proportion of doping users seem to be found at fitness centres and in gyms. Simon *et al.* (2006) have found that 12.5 per cent of the visitors of 49 fitness centres in Germany had used AAS preparations. In another study of 113 fitness centres in Germany by Striegel *et al.* (2006) the results showed that 13.5 per cent had used AAS. This is a large group of users if we consider that almost five million people visited fitness centres in Germany at the time.

Among young people, in a nationwide high school study in the USA including 15,000 respondents, Dodge and Jaccard (2006) found that 2.7 per cent of boys and 0.4 per cent of girls had used AAS. In Poland Sas-Nowosielski (2006) conducted a survey of Polish students between the ages of 15 to 22, where 9 per cent of the boys and 2 per cent of the girls reported use of AAS (cf. Rachon *et al.*, 2005). The motives for using among the Polish students were cosmetic – to achieve a more beautiful body in relation to cultural ideals of body shape. However, the use of AAS does not only exist among youth. In an internet study by Parkinson and Evans (2006) of 500 AAS users, only 2.6 per cent were teenagers and the debut age was between 20 and 24. The vast majority of respondents were men (98.8 per cent). Only a few of the respondents used AAS with a sporting motive; 78.4 per cent were not competing in bodybuilding or any other sport. The most frequent motive for using AAS was cosmetic.

Even though there are different motives for different types of doping use, there are also common dominators between doping uses in different contexts which differ from other types of substance abuse (e.g. alcohol and narcotics). Doping in society, like doping in sport, is primarily motivated by its ability to increase performance, whether it is to accomplish better results in sports competitions, to sculpt a muscular and beautiful body in a more efficient manner or to be a more efficient criminal (stronger and more fearsome).

Doping use has to be understood in its own right

Individuals who abuse alcohol or drugs, or who engage in criminality, are usually known as 'risk-taking individuals' and have been shown in several studies to have an increased predisposition for the use of doping preparations. Papadopoulos *et al.* (2006) conclude that use of doping is three times more likely among individuals who report often being intoxicated by alcohol. Wichstrøm (2006) suggests a connection between doping use and substantial alcohol consumption, drug use, early sexual activity, depression, eating disorders and suicide attempts. In a study of 16,000 high school students in the USA, Miller *et al.* (2002) showed that users of AAS were more likely to engage in other risk behaviours (cf. Kanayama *et al.*, 2010). A similar pattern is suggested in a study of 2,742 Swedish high school students; Kindlundh *et al.* (1999) found an association between the use of tobacco, alcohol and drugs and use of AAS.

The connection between risk behaviour and doping use has also been suggested in more 'sport-specific' studies. In one study, Kanayama *et al.* (2003)

compared 48 male AAS-using weightlifters with 45 non-using weightlifters. The AAS users had higher rates of illicit drug use prior to AAS use than the non-users. Thiborg and Carlsson (2007) report in a study of Swedish athletes that the doping users were more 'sensation-seeking', meaning that they were inclined to look for adventure and live on the edge to a higher degree, viewing health risks and the risk of getting caught by doping control measures as less problematic than non-users. In a study of attitudes that affect the use of doping substances, Donovan *et al.* (2002) include 'risk-taking' as a personal factor which influences attitudes in relation to doping.

Despite this evidence, questions remain about the relationship between risk behaviours and doping, and about whether the relation is valid in sport contexts as well as in other social contexts (gyms, criminal contexts, prisons etc.) and in relation to doping with other motives than sporting ones (e.g. doping for cosmetic reasons). For example, in a study of 15,000 sports participating high school students in the USA, there was no correlation between doping use and risk behaviours (Dodge and Jaccard, 2006). Coakley and Pike (2009) argue that there is a significant difference between young people using alcohol and narcotics to escape from reality and athletes using drugs to improve athletic performance. They argue that the use of doping substances does not aim to violate social and legal norms, in contrast to abusing alcohol and drugs. Use of doping preparations is rather a manifestation of an 'over conformity' in relation to sports norms – the 'sport ethic' (which not should be confused with norms of fair play). The fundamental values of sports – the 'sport ethic' – are characterized as the way athletes should prioritize sports and their team before everything else in life. The athlete should continually strive to improve sporting performances, fighting for wins and records and overcoming obstacles in the struggle for victories. Doping is a tool in that endeavour.

It is clear that risk behaviour is not sufficient to explain doping use generally. Most of the studies (although not all) which suggest risk behaviour as an explanation for the use of doping preparations are conducted on school populations rather than on specific sports groups (e.g. Kindlundh *et al.*, 1999; Miller *et al.*, 2002; Papadopoulos *et al.*, 2006; Wichstrøm, 2006). To differentiate doping use within sport from drug use (and doping use) outside sport can be relevant (cf. Coakley and Pike, 2009). It is possible that students who are using doping substances without any sporting ambitions are more risk-taking than individuals from sporting populations, such as elite-level athletes (cf. Hoff, 2013; Kanayama *et al.*, 2006; Pope *et al.*, 1997). However, this issue is probably more complex. For instance, an individual who is lifting weights every day in the gym to build strength and muscles and is using AAS without any sporting ambitions may be associated with neither risk behaviour nor sporting 'over conformity' (cf. Cohen *et al.*, 2007; Monaghan, 2001). This may reflect on a different type of doping which has nothing to do with risk, revolt, escape or competitive sport. Cohen *et al.* (2007) have shown in a study of AAS users that most of the users were not risk-taking youth or 'cheating' athletes. The typical user was instead a male, Caucasian, highly educated, gainfully employed professional, approximately 30 years old, who was earning an above-average income and was not active in organized sports. Also, Monaghan's (2001) comprehensive study of AAS users in Wales does not support the association between risk behaviours such as abuse of alcohol and narcotics and the use of AAS. AAS users in his study were avoiding alcohol, drugs and tobacco since it was bad for training (cf. Hoff, 2012). To conclude, I will stress that use of doping preparations cannot only be regarded as yet another drug problem in a risk behaviour context; doping has to be studied in its own right.

Doping use is a sign of the times

In the doping literature, the use of doping has generally been regarded as an individual problem with individual causes. The reasons for doping use have mainly been found in individual motives (e.g. to win competitions), individual socio-psychological factors (e.g. a risk-taking personality) and individual attitudes (to win at any cost) (Backhouse *et al.*, 2007; Hoff and Carlsson, 2005; Hoff, 2008). This may seem peculiar, since we know that social influences have major impacts on individual behaviour in everyday life. Doping needs to be studied not only as an individual problem, I argue; the individual behaviour has to be analysed in a historic, social and societal context. However, the importance of social processes for individuals' use of doping preparations has not been studied or problematized to any significant extent. Exceptions are research on doping outside competitive sports which have discussed connections between 'muscular body ideals of society' and the use of doping preparations (Pope *et al.*, 1999, 2000, 2001). Use of doping has also been discussed in relation to 'individualization of society' and 'medicalizations of society' (Brevik *et al.*, 2009; Hoff, 2004; Kryger Pedersen, 2003; Waddington, 2000). I will briefly discuss these three social perspectives and their contribution to the understanding of doping, especially doping outside the competitive sports context.

The muscular body ideals have a long history in Western society, back to ancient male muscular ideals (Johansson, 1998). Yang *et al.* (2005) have studied differences in bodily ideologies between West and East, in a comparative study of the USA and Europe on one hand and China (Taiwan) on the other. The authors found significant differences in bodily ideals. In the West, male muscular ideals were all-pervading. In the East the ideals were oriented towards psychological abilities like mental strength, independent thinking and courage. Pope *et al.* (1999, 2000, 2001) argue that the muscular bodily ideals in the West have been even more apparent during recent decades. These ideals must of course be considered when we are analysing use of muscle-building doping preparations like AAS.

When we look at the most common motive for the use of doping preparations outside competitive sport which emerges in the research on doping, it is to improve appearance, especially to become more muscular (see, for example, Backhouse *et al.*, 2007; Hoff, 2008; Parkinson and Evans, 2006; Rachon *et al.*, 2005; Sas-Nowosielski, 2006; Özdemir *et al.*, 2005). It is usually boys and men who want to be more muscular, in accordance with the prevailing gender order (see Bach, 2005; Connell, 2005; Kanayama *et al.*, 2006; Keane, 2005; Klein, 1993; Luciano, 2007, Pope *et al.*, 1993, 1997; cf. Johansson, 1998). But female body ideals can also be associated with doping. Different doping products classified as diet pills are popular among women (cf. Beals, 2004; Leifman *et al.*, 2011). Even more interesting is the new female training and body ideals which are connected to ideals of muscles and strength – for example, 'Strong is the new skinny' (Hoff, 2013; Kane, 2012). According to this ideal, which is frequently discussed on the internet, women should be physically fit and strong, and probably we cannot rule out women as AAS users in the future.

The individualization of society has been illuminated as a change in modern society where the individual has greater freedom but also a greater individual responsibility for his or her life (Bauman, 2001; Beck, 1998; Giddens, 1991). In the individualized society the individual has the possibility to construct and change his or her identity, and bodily changes are an effective way to change a person's identity (Johansson, 1998, 2006). In today's society there are many possibilities for individuals who want to change their bodies: for example, cosmetic surgery, tattoos, piercing, diet pills and work-outs. With this point of departure the use of doping substances can be analysed as a tool in an individual effort to construct a new identity through bodily changes, e.g. bigger muscles (Breivik *et al.*, 2009; Hoff, 2008).

Lund Kirkegaard (2007) has analysed the fast growing fitness industry in Denmark as an expression of the modern individualized society where the view that beautiful people live good lives is the ultimate selling point for fitness centres. But there is a downside to this individual freedom of constructing new identities through bodily changes: the individual also has a greater responsibility for her or his body in the modern individualized society. There is no excuse for bodies that fall outside the frame of the ideal body. The infinite methods of exercise and cosmetic surgery available leave no options for individuals who want to fit into the frame of successful lives and make it hard to neglect bodily shortcomings.

If we connect the process of individualization, where the individual has an increased interest in constructing or changing his or her body and identity at the fitness centre, in accordance with society's muscular body ideals, the interest in muscle enhancing doping substances is not difficult to grasp. Doping preparations like AAS can be used as an effective tool in the identity-changing process. The preparations can serve as a shortcut to a new life.

Medicalization of society is a discourse which started in the 1960s and analyses the meaning of the expansion of medicine in society in the second half of the twentieth century. The sociologist I.K. Zola (1972) argues that modern medicine has developed into an institution for social control within industrialized society. People become labelled by physicians as healthy or sick, i.e. 'normal' or 'abnormal'. In the discourse of medicalization these labels have moral implications. Conrad and Schneider (1992) express this process as going from badness to illness. Illich (1975) has shown how new groups in society have been put under medical surveillance, for instance the unborn, the newborn, infants, menopausal women, the elderly, rowdy schoolchildren, etc. More and more human conditions are considered to be sickness, and are put into the frame of medical 'jurisdiction', for example alcoholism and drug addiction, and today we encounter several new psychiatric diagnoses like ADHD (cf. de Swaan, 1988).

The medicalization process has also influenced sport. Waddington (2000) has analysed doping in sport as a part of sports being medicalized during the second half of the twentieth century, where the industrialized society was characterized by an increased politicization and commercialization. Doctors and drugs became crucial elements in sport to help athletes achieve improved sporting performances by offering rehabilitation, more efficient work-out methods, treatment through medications, and in some cases treatment with doping preparations. A distinct example of the importance of medicine for the development of doping in sport is the medical innovation of blood doping. The method was invented by medical researchers as a performance enhancing method which was legitimate at the time (Waddington, 2000).

Medicalization does not only influence institutions and organizations like healthcare and sport; the process is also influencing individuals. Individuals today have great faith in healthcare and drugs. Individuals also seem to embrace medical approaches when it comes solving different individual problems. With different forms of psychotropic drugs we can keep away unwanted feelings and states of mind. The huge interest in self-help methods is also probably an expression of today's medicalized and individualized society (cf. Johansson, 2006). With different forms of drugs we can increase sexual and intellectual performances. With cosmetic surgery we can improve our appearance. The exceedingly large market of dietary supplements seems to follow the same logic – quick fixes – to use a pill to solve different problems and to enhance individual performances. Using doping drugs to accomplish bodily goals is yet another phenomenon where the individual is influenced by medical thinking. In an interview study of AAS-using individuals, some of the informants represented what the author called 'the medicalized individual'. They acted as their own doctors and used different drugs to accomplish certain goals, such as bigger muscles or better endurance, or they solved problems like fatigue and insomnia with different drugs. But they were not only their own physicians; they were also behaving like medical scientists and experimented on their own bodies with different medicines in search of an effective drug which their competing bodybuilding fellows did not know about (Hoff, 2016a).

We should not only look at current social processes at societal level to understand doping behaviours: we should also look at doping behaviours from a social group perspective. What importance has the social surroundings of an individual, for example in the gym, for his or her decision to use doping substances? If doping use is a natural part of the training regime of people in the surroundings of the gym where you exercise, this will probably have an effect on your own values and behaviour in relation to doping. There are not many studies investigating this social level of reality in relation to doping, but some research results describe how values and behaviour in the social environment are important impact factors for doping use.

In a study of earlier competing powerlifters who had used AAS, their narratives were interpreted as a social learning process with a point of departure from Lave and Wenger's (1991) and Wenger's (1998) learning theories. The informants learned that others in the community were using doping substances; they learned that most of their competitors were using preparations; they learned that officials were aware of the extensive doping use and several of them had also used doping preparations in their earlier careers; they learned, often from senior lifters, about AAS – how to use the preparations and how to avoid being caught in a doping control, with the older lifters often serving as mentors both in relation to training and in relation to doping; they learned that fellow athletes in the community were assuming that they were using AAS if they were performing well; they learned that they would be questioned if they asserted that they were not using AAS; they learned that if they were to use AAS they would be a lot better; and finally they learned where to purchase AAS – and could purchase them within the powerlifting community (Hoff, 2016b; CF. Andreasson, 2014). This understanding of group dynamic processes could be transferred to other social arenas like bodybuilding communities and elite athlete communities, but also to groups of recreational gym users, youth groups or criminal groups.

The pursuit of good health could become unhealthy

What do I mean by this claim? I mean that the ideals of health, fitness and workouts in today's society are closely connected to society's body ideals, which are ideals that could lead to eating disorders and the use of doping substances; striving for better health can become unhealthy. In today's society health and workouts are in focus. In Western societies, lifestyle deaths result in huge economic costs for public healthcare, and cause individual suffering. Physical activity is demonstrably beneficial for health and for preventing both physical and mental health problems (see, for example, Aurélio *et al.*, 2005). The investment in 'exercise on prescription' in the healthcare system in some European countries is a clear consequence of this development (see, for example, Mellquist, 2006). It is healthy to exercise, it is healthy to eat less sugar and fat, but there is a limit where excessive behaviours in relation to these recommendations become unhealthy: exercise becomes an obsession and leads to unhealthily thin bodies with too low a proportion of fat, or the focus on diet becomes an exaggerated preoccupation with food and calories, resulting in eating disorders. Excessive training and dieting can also be connected to the use of different hormonal doping substances, in attempts to achieve either an extremely thin body or an extremely muscular body.

Obsessive muscle building and AAS using among men have been compared with anorexia among women. Women with anorexia see themselves as plump when they are looking at themselves in the mirror; muscle-building men using AAS see themselves as thin and small in the mirror. This latter phenomenon has been discussed as 'muscle dysmorphia' (Blouin and Goldfield, 1995; Goldfield *et al.*, 2006; Kanayama *et al.*, 2003, 2006; Pope *et al.*, 1993, 1997; cf. Keane,

2005). Both of these behaviours are probably reactions to Western body ideals, but the reactions are inverted (Pope *et al.*, 1993, 1997). However, both anorexia and muscle dysmorphia can also be connected to the ideals of health and exercise, but in an obsessive way. The connection between the health discourse and use of AAS and work-outs becomes evident in Monaghan's 2001 study, where AAS-using men considered themselves as healthy; they exercised, they were on healthy diets, they did not drink alcohol and they did not smoke.

Today's interest in health activities has grown in a high performance society. The demands in people's working lives are perceived as higher than before and stress, mental illnesses and fatigue syndromes are increasing. People find it harder to cope with the daily life, including work, children, family, friends and leisure activities. This stressful life needs a counterweight in terms of exercise and health activities. And in our consumer-oriented culture it is not enough to own new cars, designer kitchens, expensive clothes, etc. (cf. Featherstone, 2007; Slater, 1998). It is also a status symbol to 'own' a beautiful and fit body, which can be 'bought' at the fitness centre. The health trend and individuals' increased interest in physical activity fits neatly into the supply of different forms of exercise that the gym and fitness industry can supply. The fitness industry has grown exponentially during the last couple of decades (see, for example, Andreasson and Johansson, 2014; Lund Kirkegaard, 2007). Different forms of fitness workout activities, including strength training, seems to have replaced earlier more collective forms of exercise in sports clubs (Ibsen, 2006). In the individualized society, individual request individual schedules, individual training programmes and personal trainers (cf. Ibsen, 2006). Lund Kirkegaard (2007: 132) describes the process in these words:

> The central commercial element in the body's historical socialization process is that the ideal physics of the body and appearance have slowly become a commercial commodity, which can be purchased.... The perception that beautiful people live good lives stands as a faultless and efficient mantra for the commercial success of the fitness industry.
>
> (My translation)

We are here dealing with two different values: the ideal of a healthy body and the ideal of a beautiful body, and these different ideals, I argue, coincide, at least in a commercial sense. When we look at the front of different health magazines, they are often covered with beautiful, fit, muscular men or slim but fit women. If we look inside the magazines, they are filled with advertisements for different kinds of dietary supplements, like muscle-building protein powder. The logic of beauty and fitness is closely linked together. And the logic of using legal performance enhancing dietary supplements is close to the logic of using illegal doping preparations – in both cases the purpose is to enhance performance, to build muscles in a more effective and speedy manner or to slim. In the significant cases of eating disorders and of AAS-using individuals which have come into focus, we cannot ignore the impact of society's beauty ideals and ideals of fitness and health (cf. Beals, 2004; Striegel *et al.*, 2006; Simon *et al.*, 2006; Pope *et al.*, 1993, 1997, 1999, 2000, 2001). These processes influence girls and boys, women and men.

Conclusions

In this article I argue for a broader understanding of doping, and make some reflections on the subject. Doping is not only an issue for competitive sports; doping exists in several other contexts in society, and with other motives than sporting motives. The most common are to be more muscular and beautiful in a gym context, to be stronger and more fearsome in a criminal context, and as an ingredient in risk-taking behaviour together with substance abuse among adolescents. Even though there are plenty of motives for using doping preparations, I also point to a common dominator. Whether you use doping preparations for better sporting performances, a more muscular body, criminal strategic reasons or as an element in risk-taking substance abuse, it is about enhancing performance.

Even though several studies on doping have found a connection between risk behaviour like substance abuse and the use of doping preparations, the article questions this association. I believe that we should not too quickly and too easily consider doping preparations like AAS as yet another drug like narcotics, and not casually interpret the use of doping preparations as substance abuse behaviour. There are differences between doping preparations and narcotics and alcohol. Doping preparations are substances which enhance performances in the long run; narcotics and alcohol give instant euphoria and are used to escape from reality. And if we look at studies of frequent doping users, they often report an aversion to tobacco, alcohol and narcotics. While I would not dismiss the risk behaviour hypothesis as an explanation for doping use, it needs to be interrogated, and we should look also for other explanations.

Another reflection or critique of the doping research today is the lack of social perspectives on the use of doping substances. With some exceptions, research has focused solely on individual perspectives of doping use. But we cannot find the explanation for doping use only in individual motives and psycho-social backgrounds. Individuals are acting within frames of social structures and ideals. In this article I address three social perspectives which I find useful: the body ideals of society, the individualization of society and the medicalization of society. These perspectives have been discussed in doping research. Today we see a renaissance of muscular body ideals in Western society which we must of course consider as an important impact factor for the use of muscle-building preparations like AAS. The individualized society gives individuals a greater freedom to choose lifestyles and identities. And bodily changes are effective for creating identity changes. Today, individuals have infinite opportunities to alter the body, for example by cosmetic surgery, dieting, piercing, tattoos and workouts, and using doping preparations is yet another technique in that arsenal. And it is a method that fits well into our medicalized society, which is a perspective that analyses the greater importance of medicine in the industrial society, where medical treatment and drugs are influencing increasing numbers of society sectors and human conditions. The medicalization of society, I argue, is also influencing individuals in 'medical thinking'. It is becoming natural to use medical treatment and drugs to solve different problems in life and also to achieve goals like, for instance, getting a more muscular body by using doping substances.

Another social issue which I discuss in the article is the current ideal of health in today's society. This health ideal I connect with society's body ideals. Individuals probably do not only work out and eat healthier food just to improve their health. Exercise and diet regimes seem to be popular methods to control and shape modern fit bodies. And this behaviour entails risks when it becomes obsessive, in the form of both eating disorders and excessive strength-training, which can include the use of doping preparations.

These different social perspectives on doping are not only important as separate explanations of doping behaviours. The perspectives are connected and they reinforce each other, I finally argue. In the individualized society with its current muscular body ideals, individuals try to construct bodies and identities which are in accordance with these ideals. With the influences of health ideals, exercise and dieting become important. To strive for a healthy and fit (and beautiful) body is yet another important goal in society. In our consumer culture it has become a status symbol to possess a fit and perfect body. And in a 'medical era', with medical thinking and countless medical methods (e.g. cosmetic surgery, dieting) and drugs like doping preparations, it is not farfetched to understand the desire of individuals to use medical techniques and drugs in their endeavour for a new body and identity. Interestingly, in our individualized society, individuals have a freedom to (re)construct their bodies and identities and have access to infinite methods. In that respect, everyone appears to strive towards the same ideals, at least when it comes to body and appearance. The effort for a more beautiful body seems not to be one of free choice and a positive goal in individuals' lives. Instead, from the ideals of beauty, health and fitness appears to put a lot of social pressure on individuals who fall outside the frame of these ideals, which can create anxiety and an obsession in relation to bodily changes, resulting in excessive training, recurrent cosmetic surgery, obesity surgery, eating disorders and use of doping preparations. The methods and substances exist – what is your excuse for not using them when your body is 'imperfect'?

References

Andreasson, J. (2014) 'Shut up and squat!': learning body knowledge within the gym. *Etnography and Education*, 9 (1), 1–15.

Andreasson, J. and Johansson, T. (2014) The fitness revolution: historical transformations in the global gym and fitness culture. *Sport Science Review*, XXIII (3-4), 91–112.

Aurélio, M., Peluso, M. and Silviera Guerra de Andrade, L.H. (2005) Physical activity and mental health: the association between exercise and mood. *Clinics*, 60 (1), 61–70.

Bach, A.R. (2005) *Mænd och muskler: En bog om styrketæning og anabole steroider* (Men and Muscles: A Book about Strength Training and Anabolic Steroids). København: Tiderna skifter.

Backhouse, S., McKenna, J., Robinson, S. and Atkin, A. (2007) *International Literature Review: Attitudes, Behaviours, Knowledge and Education – Drugs in Sport: Past, Present and Future.* Leeds: Carnegie Research Institute.

Bauman, Z. (2001) *The Individualized Society.* Cambridge: Polity Press.

Beals, A.K. (2004) *Disordered Eating among Athletes: A Comprehensive Guide for Health Professionals.* Champaign: Human Kinetics.

Beck, U. (1998) *Risksamhället: På väg mot en annan modernitet* (Risk Society: Towards a New Modernity). Göteborg: Daidalos.

Blouin, A.G. and Goldfield, G.S. (1995) Body image and steroid use in male bodybuilders. *International Journal of Eating Disorders*, 18, 159–165.

Breivik, G., Hanstad, D.V. and Loland, S. (2009) Attitudes towards use of performance-enhancing substances and body modification techniques: a comparison between elite athletes and the general population. *Sport in Society*, 12 (6), 737–754.

Coakley, J. and Pike, E. (2009). *Sports in Society: Issues and Controversies.* London: McGraw-Hill.

Cohen, J., Collins, R., Darkes, J. and Gwartney, D. (2007) A league of their own: demographics, motivations and patterns of use of 1,955 male adult non-medical anabolic steroid users in the United States. *Journal of the International Society of Sports Nutrition*, 4 (12), doi: 10.1186/1550-2783-4-12.

Connell, R.W. (2005) *Masculinities.* Cambridge: Polity Press.

Conrad, P. and Schneider, J.W. (1992) *Deviance and Medicalization: From Badness to Sickness.* Philadelphia: Temple.

de Swaan, A. (1988) *In the Care of the State.* Cambridge: Polity Press.

Dodge, T.L. and Jaccard, J.J. (2006) The effect of high school sports participation on the use of performance-enhancing substances in young adulthood. *Journal of Adolescent Health*, 39, 367–373.

Donovan, R.J., Egger, G., Kapernick, V. and Mendoza, J. (2002) A conceptual framework for achieving performance enhancing drug compliance in sport. *Sports Medicine*, 32, 269–284.

Featherstone, M. (2007) *Consumer Culture and Postmodernism.* London: Sage.

Giddens, A. (1991) *Modernity and Self-identity: Self and Society in the Late Modern Age.* Cambridge: Polity Press.

Goldfield, G.S., Blouin, A.G. and Woodside, D.B. (2006) Body image, binge eating, and bulimia nervosa in male bodybuilders. *Canadian Journal of Psychiatry*, 51 (3), 160–168.

Hermansson, G. and Moberg, T. (2008) *Anabola androgena steroider 1.1* (Anabolic Androgenic Steroids 1.1). Göteborg: Mediahuset.

Hoff, D. (2004) Sociala styrningsformer och antidopningspolicy – en rättssociologisk forskningsstrategi tillämpad på antidopningsarbetet inom idrotten (Social governance and anti-doping policy: a sociology of law research strategy applied on the anti-doping work in sports). Idrottsforum.org (ISSN 1652–7224).

Hoff, D. (2008) Doping- och antidopingforskning: en inventering av samhälls- och beteendevetenskaplig forskning och publikationer 2004–2007. (Doping and Anti-doping Research: An Inventory of Social and Behavioural Research and Publications 2004–2007). FoU-rapport 2008:1. Stockholm: Riksidrottsförbundet.

Hoff, D. (2012) Doping, risk and abuse: an interview study of elite athletes with a history of steroid use. *Performance Enhancement and Health*, 1 (2), 61–65.

Hoff, D. (2013) Dopning utanför idrotten – Individualisering och muskulösa skönhetsideal: en studie i grundskola, gymnasium och på gym i Kalmar (Doping outside sports – individualisation and muscular beauty ideals: a study of elementary schools, high schools and fitness centres in Kalmar municipality). *Scandinavian Sport Studies Forum*, 4, 1–24.

Hoff, D. (2016a) Dopningens olika ansikten: En kvalitativ studie av AAS-användning på gym. (Different faces of doping: A qualitative study of AAS use at gyms.) Research Reports in Social Work 2016:1. Lund: School of Social Work, Lund University.

Hoff, D. (2016b) The significance of social learning processes for doping use in the elite sport environment: An interview study of AAS-using powerlifters. (Article manuscript.)

Hoff, D. and Carlsson, B. (2005) *Doping- och antidopingforskning: En rättssociologisk inventering av samhälls- och beteendevetenskaplig forskning och publikationer* (Doping and Anti-doping Research: A Sociology of Law Inventory of Social and Behavioural Research and Publications). FoU-rapport 2005:1. Stockholm: Riksidrottsförbundet.

Ibsen, B. (2006) *Foreningsidrætten i Danmark: Udvikling og udfordringar.* (Sport Associations in Denmark: Development and Challenges). Köpenhavn: Idrættens Analyseinstitut.

Illich, I. (1975) *Medical Nemesis.* London: Calder & Boyars.

Johansson, P., Lindqvist, A.-S., Nyberg, F. and Fahlke, C. (2000) Anabolic androgenic steroids affects alcohol intake, defensive behaviors and brain opioid peptides in the rat. *Pharmacology Biochemistry and Behavior*, 67, 271–279.

Johansson, T. (1998) *Den skulpterade kroppen: Gymkultur, friskvård och estetik* (The Sculptured Body: Gym Culture, Prophylaxis and Aesthetics). Stockholm: Carlssons Bokförlag.

Johansson, T. (2006) *Makeovermani: Om Dr Phil, plastkirurgi och illusionen om det perfekta jaget* (Makeover Mania: About Dr Phil, Cosmetic Surgery and the Illusion of the Perfect Self). Stockholm: Natur och Kultur.

Kanayama, G., Barry, S. and Hudson, J.I. (2006) Body image and attitudes toward male roles in anabolic-androgenic steroid users. *American Journal of Psychiatry*, 163, 697–703.

Kanayama, G., Brower, K.J., Wood, R.I., Hudson, J.I. and Pope, H.G. (2010) Treatment of anabolic-androgenic steroid dependence: emerging evidence and its implications. *Drug and Alcohol Dependence*, 109, 6–13.

Kanayama, G., Pope, H.G., Cohane, G. and Hudson, J.I. (2003) Risk factors for anabolic androgenic steroid use among weightlifters. *Drug and Alcohol Dependence*, 71, 77–86.

Kane, J. (2012) Can strong really be the new skinny? *Journal of Psychical Education, Recreation and Dance*, 83 (6), 6–12.

Keane, H. (2005) Diagnosing the male steroid user: drug use, body image and disordered masculinity. *Health*, 9 (2), 189–208.

Kindlundh, A.M., Isacson, D.G., Berglund, L. and Nyberg, F. (1999) Factors associated with adolescent use of doping agents: anabolic-androgenic steroids. *Addiction*, 94, 543–553.

Klein, A. (1993) *Little Big Men: Bodybuilding Subculture and Gender Construction.* Albany: State University of New York Press.

Kryger Pedersen, I. (2003) Lægemidlers indtog i sport og motion (The entry of drugs in sports and exercise). *Social Kritik*, 15 (90), 24–35.

Lave, J. and Wenger, E. (1991) *Situated Learning: Legitimate Peripheral Participation.* Cambridge: Cambridge University Press.

Leifman, H., Rehnman, C., Sjöblom, E. and Holgersson, S. (2011) Anabolic androgenic steroids – use and correlates among gym users: an assessment study using questionnaires and observations at gyms in the Stockholm region. *International Journal of Environmental Research and Public Health*, 8 (7), 2656–2674.

Lindqvist, A.-S., Johansson-Steensland, P., Nyberg, F. and Fahlke, C. (2002) Anabolic androgenic steroid affects competitive behaviour, behavioural response to ethanol and brain serotonin levels. *Behavioural Brain Research*, 133, 21–29.

Luciano, L. (2007) Muscularity and masculinity in the United States: a historical overview, in J.K. Thompson and G. Cafri (eds) *The Muscular Ideal: Psychological, Social, and Medical Perspectives.* Washington: APA.

Lund Kirkegaard, K. (2007) *Fra muskelmasse til massebevægelse: Indblik i den kommercielle fitness-sektors historie* (From Muscle Mass to Mass Movement: Insight into the Commercial Fitness Sector's History). København: Idrettens Analyseinstitut.

Mellquist, A. (2006) *Fysisk aktivitet på recept (FaR): Perspektiv från idrottsrörelsen lokalt och regionalt* (Exercise on Prescription: Perspectives on Sports Movements Locally and Regionally). Stockholm: Riksidrottsförbundet, FoU-rapport 2006:3.

Mickelsson, K. (2009) *Dopningen i Sverige – en inventering av utbredning, konsekvenser och åtgärder* (Doping in Sweden: An Inventory of Spread, Consequences and Measures). Östersund: Statens folkhälsoinstitut, Rapport 2009:15.

Miller, K.E., Barnes, G.M., Sabo, D., Melnick, M.J. and Farrell, M.P. (2002) A comparison of health risk behaviour in adolescent users of anabolic androgenic steroids, by gender and athlete status. *Sociology of Sport Journal*, 19, 385–402.

Moberg, T. and Hermansson, G. (2006) *Mandom, mod och morske män: Anabola androgena steroider – Medicinskt, rättsligt och socialt* (Manhood, Courage, and Tough Men: Anabolic Androgenic Steroids – Medical, Legal and Social Perspectives). Göteborg: Mediahuset.

Monaghan, L.F. (2001) *Bodybuilders, Drugs and Risk.* New York: Routledge.

Özdemir, L., Nur, N., Bagcivan, I., Bulut, O., Sümer, H. and Tezeren, G. (2005) Doping and performance enhancing drug use in athletes living in Sivas, mid-Anatolia: a brief report. *Journal of Sports Science and Medicine*, 4 (3), 248–252.

Papadopoulos, F.C., Skalkidis, I., Parkkar, J. and Petridou, E. (2006) Doping use among tertiary education students in six developed countries. *European Journal of Epidemiology*, 21, 307–313.

Parkinson, A.B. and Evans, N.A. (2006) Anabolic androgenic steroids: a survey of 500 users. *Medicine and Science in Sport and Exercise*, 38 (4), 644–651.

Pope, H.G., Katz, D.L. and Hudson, J.I. (1993) Anorexia nervosa and 'reverse anorexia' among 108 male bodybuilders. *Comprehensive Psychiatry*, 34, 406–409.

Pope, H.G., Olivardia, R. and Borowiecki, J.J. (1999) Evolving ideals of male body image as seen through action toys. *International Journal of Eating Disorder*, 26 (1), 65–72.

Pope, H.G., Phillips K.A. and Olivardia, R. (2000) *The Adonis Complex: The Secret Crisis of Male Body Obsession.* New York: Free Press.

Pope, H.G., Phillips, K.A. and Olivardia, R. (2001) The commercial value of male body: a longitudinal survey of advertising in women's magazines. *Psychotherapy and Psychosomatics*, 70 (4), 189–192.

Pope, H.G., Gruber, A.J., Choi, P., Olivardia, R. and Phillips, K.A. (1997) Muscle dysmorphia: an underrecognized form of body dysmorphic disorder. *Psychosomatics*, 38, 548–557.

Rachon, D., Pokrywka, L. and Suchecka-Rachon, K. (2005) Prevalence and risk factors of anabolic-androgenic steroids (AAS) abuse among adolescents and young adults in Poland. *Sozial- und Praventivmedizin*, 51 (6), 392–398.

Sas-Nowosielski, K. (2006) The abuse of anabolic-androgenic steroids by Polish school-aged adolescents. *Biology of Sport*, 23 (3), 225–235.

Simon, P., Striegel, H., Aust, F., Dietz, K. and Ulrich, R. (2006) Doping in fitness sports: estimated number of unreported cases and individual probability of doping. *Addiction*, 101 (11), 1640–1644.

Skårberg, K. (2009) *Anabolic Androgenic Steroid Users in Treatment: Social Background, Drug Use Patterns, and Criminality*. Örebro: Örebro University.

Slater, D. (1998) *Consumer Culture and Modernity*. Cambridge: Polity Press.

Striegel, H., Simon, P., Frisch, S., Roeker, K., Dietz, K., Dickhuth, H.H. and Ulrich, R. (2006) Anabolic ergogenic substance users in fitness-sports: a distinct group supported by the health care system. *Drug and Alcohol Dependence*, 81 (1), 11–19.

Thiblin, I. and Pärlklo, T. (2002) Anabolic androgenic steroids and violence. *Acta Psychiatrica Scandinavica*, 106, 125–128.

Thiborg, J. and Carlsson, B. (2007) *Doping: Personlighet, motiv och moral i idrotten* (Doping: Personality, Motives and Morals in Sport). Stockholm: Riksidrottsförbundet, Rapport 2007: 10.

Waddington, I. (2000) *Sport, Health and Drugs: A Critical Sociological Perspective*. London: E. & F.N. Spon.

Wenger, E. (1998) *Communities of Practice: Learning, Meaning, and Identity*. Cambridge: Cambridge University Press.

Wichstrøm, L. (2006) Predictors of future anabolic androgenic steroid use. *Medicine and Science in Sports and Exercise*, 38, 1578–1583.

Yang, C.F.J., Gray, P. and Pope, H.G. (2005) Male body image in Taiwan versus the West: Yanggang Zhiqi meets the adonis complex. *American Journal of Psychiatry*, 162 (2), 263–269.

Zola, I.K. (1972) Medicine as an institution of social control. *Sociological Review*, 20, 487–504.

5 Adulterated nutritional supplements and unapproved pharmaceuticals as new sources of doping substances for fitness and recreational sports

Hans Geyer

During the past years, two new sources of doping substances aiming predominantly at fitness and recreational sports have been identified: The markets for adulterated nutritional supplements and for unapproved pharmaceuticals.

Adulterated nutritional supplements – introduction

Within the market of adulterated nutritional supplements, particularly products containing stimulants, anabolic steroids and/or β_2-agonists have been detected. Noteworthy, these pharmacologically active substances have not been declared on the list of ingredients. These classes of drugs are categorized as doping agents by the World Anti-Doping Agency (WADA) and are only available, if at all, on prescription. The adulterated supplements are commonly advertised with the effects of the undeclared pharmaceuticals such as fat loss, muscle growth, neuro-enhancement, and increased training motivation (training booster). The substances are admixed to the nutritional supplements in therapeutic or even supra-therapeutic doses and are connected with severe health risks. Therefore medical doctors treating unexplainable health problems of fitness enthusiasts and recreational athletes should also take into consideration that health issues may arise from the unintentional consumption of pharmacologically active doping agents via nutritional supplements.

Nutritional supplements adulterated with stimulants

Currently, the main stimulants found as adulterants of nutritional supplements are ephedrine and its analogues, sibutramine, methylhexaneamine oxilofrine, and new "designer" stimulants such as 1,3-dimethylbutylamine or different phenylethylamines (e.g., β-methylphenylethylamine, BMPEA). Products enriched with these substances are mainly advertised as fat burner, mood enhancer, or training booster and their use has been reported in the context of adverse analytical findings in sport as well as medical emergencies.

In the case of supplements containing ephedrines, the natural sources of ephedrine such as *Ma Huang* or *ephedra sinica* are frequently mentioned on the label rather than the names of the active ingredients ephedrine, pseudoephedrine, methylephedrine, etc.

Containers of supplements enriched with sibutramine do not declare the drug on the label and the consumer is only provided with the information that the product contains "pure herbal ingredients" that are advertised to have considerable weight-loss capabilities. Sibutramine can be found in therapeutic or even supra-therapeutic doses in slimming capsules, powders and slimming teas. Sibutramine is a synthetic anorectic drug, only approved as a pharmaceutical preparation and only available on prescription. Because of its enormous side effects (stroke and heart attack risk for patients with a history of cardiovascular disease), the European Medicines Agency (EMEA) recommended the withdrawal of the drug from the market in 2010. Sibutramine has been on the WADA list of prohibited substances since 2006.

Since 2008/2009, there has been a high risk of inadvertent doping with the stimulant methylhexaneamine, which was added to the WADA Prohibited List in 2009. The issue of inadvertent doping arises from the fact that numerous different names for methylhexaneamine can be found on the label, such as dimethylamylamine, dimethylpentylamine, pentylamine, geranamine, forthane, 2-amino-4-methylhexane, etc. On WADA's 2011 Prohibited List, only the names methylhexaneamine and dimethylpentylamine are mentioned in the group of stimulants, which complicates the identification of the substance as a prohibited compound. In some supplements, geranium root extract or geranium oil is mentioned as an alleged natural source of methylhexanemine. However, recent investigations have shown that geranium does not contain methylhexaneamine, or only extremely small amounts, which means that synthetic methylhexanemine must have been added. Despite warnings by different national anti-doping agencies in 2009 and 2010, numerous elite athletes have been tested positive for methylhexaneamine in competition. In the years 2010–2014 methylhexanemanine was the most frequently detected stimulant in elite sports.

Other stimulants which can be found in adulterated nutritional supplements are oxilofrine (also known as methylsynephrine, hydroxyephrine and oxyephrine), and new designer stimulants, as for instance 1,3-dimethylbutylamine (normethylhexanamine) or phenylethylamines such as BMPEA. Supplements containing these stimulants are advertised as slimming products and training boosters. The new designer stimulants have never been tested for their efficacy and for potential adverse effects in humans.

Nutritional supplements adulterated with anabolic steroids

Since 2002, several dietary supplements have appeared on the market which are probably intentionally spiked with high amounts (more than 1 mg/g) of anabolic steroids, not declared or declared with non-approved or fancy names on the label. Among these, steroids including stanozolol, metandienone, dehydrochloromethyltestosterone, and oxandrolone have been identified. All of these steroidal agents are orally available drugs due to their 17-alkyl group, and dietary supplements containing these compounds claim effects such as an enormous enhancement of strength and lean body mass. The concentrations of the anabolic androgenic steroids were found in the therapeutic or supra-therapeutic range per serving, leading to adverse analytical findings detectable for several days and weeks respectively, depending on the type of steroid administered.

Since 2002 so-called "designer steroids" have also been used for the adulteration of nutritional supplements. These steroids are neither listed as ingredient in any currently available medication nor do their names appear in the WADA list of prohibited substances. Most of these "designer steroids" were synthesized in the 1960s and were tested only in animal studies for their anabolic and androgenic effects. Nowadays these steroidal agents are produced exclusively for the nutritional supplement market and are advertised for their anabolic or aromatase inhibiting capacities. With regard to the effects and side effects of these steroids for humans, limited or no knowledge exists. Also here, in most cases, the labelling of these products presents non-approved or fancy names of steroids. More than 40 of such designer steroids have been detected so far. The detection of metabolites of such steroids in an athlete's urine sample is likely to lead to an adverse analytical finding.

Nutritional supplements adulterated with β_2-agonists

In addition to the aforementioned issue of stimulants and anabolic androgenic steroids, nutritional supplements adulterated with supra-therapeutic doses of the β_2-agonist clenbuterol were identified that also did not declare the synthetic and pharmacologically active ingredient on the label. The supplements in question were advertised as weight-loss products, bearing the risk of severe side effects due to the extreme concentration of clenbuterol in these products (accounting for approximately 100 times the commonly recommended therapeutic dose). Because WADA has classified clenbuterol as anabolic agent, its detection in doping controls may lead to severe sanctions.

How to deal with the problem of adulterations of nutritional supplements

According to our experience, the risk of inadvertent doping is predominantly connected to dietary supplements aggressively marketed for their physiological effects, e.g., muscle gain, fat loss, and neuro-enhancement, but cannot be reduced exclusively to such products. Therefore, athletes should carefully consider the risks and benefits of dietary supplements in general. If supplementation appears essential to the athlete's diet, athletes are advised to purchase dietary supplements only from low-risk sources. Such sources are established in some countries such as Germany (www.colognelist.com), the Netherlands (http://antidoping.nl/nzvt), the UK (www.hfl.co.uk), and the US (www.nsf.org/certified/dietary), where databases list dietary supplements from companies whose products undergo frequent quality controls concerning the presence of doping agents.

However, these sources cannot guarantee that dietary supplements are free of risk, but offer a risk minimization. Dietary supplements produced by pharmaceutical companies might represent an alternative as such products have not yet been found to be contaminated with doping substances.

Unapproved pharmaceuticals – introduction

The black market of unapproved pharmaceuticals which are in or discontinued from pre-clinical or clinical trials also appears to represent a growing source of doping agents for the fitness enthusiast and recreational athlete. These substances are often advertised with the performance-enhancing effects they have exerted in pre-clinical trials with animal models. The compounds in question are advertised with anabolic, fat-reducing and anti-catabolic effects and improvements in endurance performance and regeneration. Neither the performance-enhancing effects of these substances nor their side effects in humans are fully clarified. The continuously increasing number of Internet providers offering unapproved substances, and especially confiscations by police and customs authorities, indicate a growing demand. Doping cases with GW1516, SARMs, GHRPs and HIF stabilizers have provided additional evidence that unapproved pharmaceuticals are misused in sport long before the clinical trials are completed.

Unapproved pharmaceuticals with anabolic effects

Among these pharmaceuticals the selective androgen receptor modulators (SARMs) and so-called designer steroids have the greatest potential of misuse for fitness and recreational sports.

Being categorized as "other anabolic agents," SARMs have been prohibited according to WADA's regulations since 2008. Owing to their proven anabolic properties and ability to stimulate the androgen receptor in muscle and bone, a substantial misuse potential was identified. This might be even more fueled by the fact that SARMs inhibit androgen receptor activity in other organs (e.g., skin and prostate) and have demonstrated less (or at least other) undesirable effects on the human organism than anabolic androgenic steroids. The number of new drug (or chemical) entities with SARM-like properties has been growing constantly; however, full clinical approval has not been accomplished for any of the drug candidate SARMs yet.

Although not yet approved, various kinds of SARMs, such as Andarine, Ostarine, LGD-2226, ACP-105, etc., are advertised and offered by Internet-based suppliers and are easily available. To meet legal requirements these pharmaceuticals are labeled "for research only" or "not for human use."

Designer steroids (see also the section above headed "Nutritional supplements adulterated with anabolic steroids") with assumed (or proven) anabolic–androgenic properties have become a predominant issue for doping control laboratories since the early 2000s. These compounds are not approved therapeutics and, largely, have also not undergone clinical trials. One of the first designer steroids detected in a nutritional supplement was 3β-hydroxyandrost-4-ene-7,17-dione. The most public attention, however, was received by the substance tetrahydrogestrinone (THG), which was detected in connection with the BALCO case in 2003. From 2002 until now, a total of about 40 steroidal compounds were identified by WADA-accredited laboratories. The reason for this increase of designer steroids on the black market was that prohormones and "traditional" anabolic steroids were prohibited as ingredients of nutritional supplements by a newly established law in the US, the Anabolic Steroid Control Act, which was launched in 2004. The designer steroids were not included on the list of this Control Act. The sources for such designer steroids are, among others, often Internet-based companies with Chinese addresses. These substances are easily available and are difficult for the Customs authorities to detect, as the delivery boxes are often misleading and/or products are well hidden and protected in rather creative packaging. A legal reaction to the growing black market for designer steroids is a new law in the US, the Designer Anabolic Steroid Control Act of 2014.

Unapproved pharmaceuticals with endurance performance-enhancing effects

Based on confiscation data of custom and police authorities and positive findings in doping controls, the main candidates among unapproved pharmaceuticals which may be misused for the enhancement of endurance performance in fitness and recreational sports are HIF-stabilizers, the AMPK agonist AICAR and the PPARδ agonist GW1516.

The use of HIF (hypoxia inducible factor) stabilizers leads to a stimulation of the endogenous EPO production by mimicking a reduced oxygen tension. The main advantage of these compounds over approved erythropoiesis stimulating agents (ESAs) such as EPO and its second- and third-generation successors is their oral availability and lack of concerns about immunogenicity. Substances of this group as FG-4592 and FG-2216 are available via Internet-based providers.

GW1516, a drug developed for the treatment of metabolic disorders and obesity, has been shown to lead to an enhancement of endurance performance. The combination of exercise and pharmacological stimulation of the PPARδ receptor using GW1516 yielded significantly enhanced physical performance (longer distance and period of running), which was increased by approximately 70 percent. The performance enhancement is based on a increased mitochondriogenesis and an improved fat utilization. Contrary to this drug, the AMPK agonist AICAR does not need an exercise stimulus to trigger an increased mitochondriogenesis and an improved fat utilization. AICAR was confiscated in huge amounts from team doctors in cycling during major events.

For all these substances neither their effects nor their side effects are fully explored yet.

Unapproved substances with growth hormone-related effects

To this group belong growth hormone secretagogues (GHS), growth hormone releasing hormones (GHRHs), and growth hormone releasing peptides (GHRPs).

All these substances stimulate the human growth hormone secretion (hGH) by different routes of action and received an enormous stimulus for illicit and mostly Internet-based sales in connection with aims of anti-aging, weight loss and muscle growth. In particular, GHS and some GHRPs have gained high popularity because of their oral bioavailability. Some of the pharmaceuticals of this group are approved (e.g., the GHRHs tesamorelin and sermorelin; GHRP-2, pralmorelin) but research concerning new potent analogs of such pharmaceuticals as therapeutic agents has been continued uninterruptedly for decades. Unapproved pharmaceuticals, which are available on the black market and are found in confiscations, are e.g., the GHRHs CJC-1295, the GHRPs GHRP-4, GHRP-6, Hexarelin, Alexamorelin, Ipamorelin, etc.

Further unapproved pharmaceuticals with doping relevance

Further unapproved substances, which may be misused in elite as well as amateur sport and are on the radar of preventive anti-doping research are: Sirtuin-1 activators, Ryanodine receptor-calstabin-complex stabilizers (Rycals) such as S107, phosphodiesterase-4 (PDE4) inhibitors, small interfering RNA (SiRNA), oligonucleotides, and myostatin-inhibitors.

Conclusion

New sources of doping substances are the market of adulterated nutritional supplements and unapproved pharmaceuticals. These are extremely fast-growing markets because of the readily available raw materials needed for doping substances and the ease of trading the products via the Internet.

The use of substances from both sources may be connected with severe health risks. Therefore medical doctors treating unexplainable health problems in fitness enthusiasts and recreational athletes should also take into consideration that health issues may be due to the consumption of doping substances via adulterated nutritional supplements or unapproved pharmaceuticals.

For the near future, new supplements adulterated with new designer stimulants for weight loss and neuro-enhancement, with diuretics for fast weight loss, with antidepressants for neuro-enhancement and with new SARMs and designer steroids for muscle growth can be expected. First findings on supplements adulterated with the antidepressant fluoxetine and with diuretics have been reported.

References

Geyer, H., Braun, H., Burke, L.M., Stear, S.J., and Castell, L.M. Inadvertent doping. In: A–Z of nutritional supplements: dietary supplements, sports nutrition foods and ergogenic aids for health and performance – Part 22. *Br. J. Sports Med.* 2011; 45: 752–754.

Geyer, H., Parr, M.K., Mareck, U., Reinhart, U., Schrader, Y., and Schänzer, W. Analysis of non-hormonal nutritional supplements for anabolic-androgenic steroids – results of an international study. *Int. J. Sports Med.* 2004; 25: 124–129.

Geyer, H., Parr, M.K., Koehler, K., Mareck, U., Schänzer, W., and Thevis, M. Nutritional supplements cross-contaminated and faked with doping substances. *J. Mass. Spectrom.* 2008; 43: 892–902.

Geyer, H., Schänzer, W., and Thevis, M. Anabolic agents: recent strategies for their detection and protection from inadvertent doping. *Br. J. Sports Med.* 2014 (May); 48 (10): 820–826.

Kohler, M., Thomas, A., Geyer, H., Petrou, M., Schänzer, W., and Thevis, M. Confiscated black market products and nutritional supplements with non-approved ingredients analyzed in the Cologne doping control laboratory 2009. *Drug Test Analysis* 2010 (November); 2 (11–12): 533–537.

Krug, O., Thomas, A., Walpurgis, K., Piper, T., Sigmund, G., Schänzer, W., Laussmann, T., and Thevis, M. Identification of black market products and potential doping agents in Germany 2010–2013. *Eur. J. Clin. Pharmacol.* 2014; 70: 1303–1311.

Thevis, M. and Schänzer, W. Emerging drugs – potential for misuse in sport and doping control detection strategies. *Mini-Reviews in Medicinal Chemistry* 2007; 7: 533–539.

Thevis, M. and Schänzer, W. Analytical approaches for the detection of emerging therapeutics and non-approved drugs in human doping controls. *J. Pharm. Biomed. Anal.* 2014; 101: 66–83.

Thevis, M., Geyer, H., Kamber, M., and Schänzer, W. Detection of the arylpropionamide-derived selective androgen receptor modulator (SARM) S-4 (Andarine) in a black-market product. *Drug Test Analysis* 2009; 1: 387–392.

Thevis, M., Schrader, Y., Thomas, A., Sigmund, G., Geyer, H., and Schänzer, W. Analysis of confiscated black market drugs using chromatographic and mass spectrometric approaches. *J. Anal. Toxicol.* 2008; 32: 232–240.

Thevis, M., Thomas, A., Kohler, M., Beuck, S., and Schänzer, W. Emerging drugs: mechanism of action, mass spectrometry and doping control analysis. *J. Mass Spectrom.* 2009; 44: 442–460.

6 The market for doping products

A quasi-illegal market and its suppliers

Letizia Paoli

Throughout the Western world there is a substantial demand for and supply of performance- and image-enhancing substances, ranging from anabolic steroids to stimulants, from erythropoietin (EPO) to growth hormone and many others. These are also known as "doping substances," as many are used by athletes to enhance their performance – a use that has been prohibited under sporting rules since the 1960s (Houlihan, 2002; Henne, 2009) and is also criminalized in several countries, including Italy and Sweden (Houlihan and García, 2012). For practical reasons, I use the term "doping substances" in the rest of this chapter; consider also performance-enhancing (i.e., doping) methods, such as blood transfusion); and refer to both doping substances and methods as "products."

The use of doping products has been studied in some detail. We have a reasonable understanding of why athletes, sporting, and non-sporting people increasingly use doping products, including the underlying societal factors (Pope *et al.*, 2000; Hoberman, 2005, Waddington and Smith, 2009). Several studies have attempted to estimate the prevalence of the use of some of these substances within specific groups (e.g., Striegel *et al.*, 2010) and at the national level (Paoli and Donati, 2014); for anabolic steroids, the group of substances most frequently used, epidemiological studies have been conducted (e.g., McCabe *et al.*, 2007; Kokkevi *et al.*, 2008).

Much less is known, though, about the supply-side of the "market"; indeed, the delivery of doping products to users and specifically athletes is not often framed as occurring in a market. Only a small number of studies have addressed the suppliers of doping products (e.g., Koert and van Kleij, 1998; Donati, 2007; Kraska *et al.*, 2010; Fincoeur and Paoli, 2014; Paoli and Donati, 2014) and criminology, as a discipline, has only recently "discovered" the topic (Paoli, 2012). Yet, the trade and distribution of doping products is subject to restrictions and prohibitions, at least in elite sport, in most European countries (Houlihan and García, 2012).

In recent years, moreover, a number of high-level international sports officials have emphasized the growing presence of the underworld in sport. David Howman, Director General of the World Anti-Doping Agency (WADA), has repeatedly denounced "the ever-increasing advance of the underworld into sport," adding that

> the underworld was making a lot of money from trafficking and distributing prohibited substances ... and that the same people who were making a lot of money out of the trafficking of prohibited substances were also making money out of illegal betting and general corruption around the fringes of sport.
>
> (WADA, 2010)

Likewise, Jacques Rogge, President of the International Olympic Committee for over ten years until 2013, repeatedly warned of the danger posed by organized crime, albeit with regard to match-fixing: "These are mafia links and mafia people and they bet at the same time while manipulating the result of a match" (e.g., Schlink, 2011). In stressing the advance of the underworld, these officials also refer to the well-publicized operations against the trade in steroids carried out by the US DEA (e.g., 2007) and a few other law enforcement agencies (e.g., Bundeskriminalamt, 2011).

Against this background, I consider the extent to which this analysis is applicable to the Italian market for doping products (in brief, "doping market"). More generally, I analyze the supply-side of the Italian market, by revisiting and building on central findings of a study on the Italian doping market conducted by Paoli and Donati (2014). On this basis, I conceptualize the doping market as a "quasi-illegal" market. It is a "market," because doping substances, if not methods, are regularly produced and exchanged – that is, distributed through complex distribution chains and sold to final users – under conditions of competition. (See Beckert and Wehinger, 2013, for a discussion of the market concept that I have brought to this analysis.) It is "quasi-illegal" because the market for doping products is being criminalized but cannot become fully illegal, as it also involves fully legal products, including life-saving medicines. An exchange or transaction involving a doping product might be fully legal, fully illegal, partly legal and illegal, or "contestable," depending on the context, including the location of the event or characteristics of the final users.

The chapter contributes to the literature on illegal markets in three ways: it represents the first systematic, empirical analysis of a national doping market, i.e., the Italian doping market; it provides a starting point for the analysis of markets for doping products in countries other than Italy; and it emphasizes the "quasi-illegality" or the often unclear, contested, and "variable" legal status of exchanges involving like doping products and, on this basis, calls for a more thorough reflection on the concept of "illegal market" and a more nuanced categorization of the various types of illegal and quasi-illegal markets.

The chapter is structured as follows. Section 6.1 describes the study research design, including the data collection; sections 6.2 and 6.3 identify the main characteristics of the suppliers of doping products in Italy and develop a typology based on their profession or occupation. Section 6.4 analyzes the distribution chains of doping products and the relationships suppliers build with each other and with users, including their use of violence and corruption. Section 6.5 singles out a unique characteristic of the elite segment of the market, typical of the recent past:

namely, the once-common protection – and, occasionally, direct involvement – of civil servants and government representatives, active in national sports bodies. Section 6.6 specifically considers the role of southern Italian mafia groups in the Italian doping market and the extent to which other actors, outside those groups, can be considered as participants in a form of organized crime. On the basis of this analysis, section 6.7 conceptualizes the doping market as a quasi-illegal market and briefly discusses the policy implications of this conceptualization.

6.1 Research design

In this chapter, I rely on the same sources of data that Paoli and Donati (2014) analyzed for the completion of their study *The Sport Doping Market: Understanding Supply and Demand and the Challenges of Their* Control, much of which was collected in close collaboration with the Carabinieri Command for Health Protection, a unit of the Italian Arma dei Carabinieri specializing in health issues. This unit is still known – and will be referred to here – with the acronym NAS from its original name, Nuclei Anti-Sofisticazione.

Our first source of information was a database with summary data for the 80 major anti-doping investigations conducted by NAS between 1999 and 2009, which represent the vast majority of the anti-doping criminal investigations and the related criminal proceedings initiated in Italy. I refer to this source as the "NAS Investigations database."

In addition to the summaries of the proceedings contained in the database, Paoli and Donati (2014) analyzed official documents related to 46 different criminal investigations; 36 of them had been carried out by NAS and were thus included in the NAS database; ten had been conducted by other police forces and were new. In some cases, the documents analyzed were the extensive summaries of the investigations written by NAS officers and submitted to the Prosecutor's Office; in other cases, the charges pressed by the prosecutors, the arrest warrants issued by the judges for preliminary investigations, or first-, second- or third-degree verdicts. I refer to these cases generically as "investigations" (from NAS's perspective) or "proceedings" (from a judicial perspective) or with the specific name of the document (e.g., verdict, charges).

Paoli and Donati (2014) also interviewed 26 NAS officers at the headquarters and in nine branch offices, as well as seven prosecutors, one policy-maker, and one other expert.[1]

Paoli and Donati also worked with various other published and unpublished materials. Among the former, they examined the annual reports of Italy's main anti-doping commission (e.g., Ministero della Salute and Istituto Superiore di Sanità, 2012) and the seizure statistics of the Italian customs agency and tax police. Lastly, they conducted an extensive review of doping-related media reports from the three main Italian news agencies – *Ansa*, *Agi*, and *Adnkronos* – for the period January 1998 through February 2012.

To strengthen our conclusions, I, as Paoli and Donati, triangulated the findings from the different sources, including an extensive media analysis.

6.2 The general characteristics of the suppliers of doping products

At risk of oversimplification, the above-mentioned criminal justice sources represent the illegal suppliers of doping products as mostly male, Italian citizens and rarely appearing to have criminal records. With few exceptions, such as the hijackers who steal doping substances from trucks, most suppliers also appear to have a legitimate profession or occupation (see Table 6.1).

Here, I highlight and discuss major findings from Table 6.1:

- Gym owners, gym managers, or body-building instructors constitute the largest category of suspects targeted by NAS investigations. Their rank reflects the persistent focus of NAS investigations on body-building and, more generally, the fitness world. In total, 158 such individuals were reported as traders in doping products in 28 of the 71 supply-related investigations contained in the NAS Investigations Database. In one of these 28 and nine other cases, an unspecified number of gym owners, managers, or instructors were also reported to be involved.
- The second largest category of suspects is associated with the world of horseracing. One large scale investigation involved 140 veterinary

Table 6.1 Leading relevant professions of the suspects reported in the NAS Investigation Database – 1999–2011

Profession	*Number of suspects reported*	*Other suspects reported, number unspecified*
Gym owners or managers and body-building instructors	158	Yes[a]
Veterinary physicians, breeders, horse drivers	140	Yes[b]
Owners or managers of dietary supplement shops	64	No
Pharmacists	20	Yes[c]
Physicians	17	Yes[d]
Staff members of cycling teams	12	Yes[e]
Sports federation officials	10	No
Law enforcement and military staff	10	No
Hospital employees	10	No
Employees and salesmen of (para-)pharmaceutical companies	6	Yes[f]
Staff of private security companies	2	No

Source: our calculations on the basis of the Database on NAS Investigations.

Notes
a In ten other investigations;
b In another investigation;
c In five other investigations;
d In three other investigations;
e In two other investigations;
f In one other investigation.

physicians, breeders and horse drivers. (Twenty-five individuals were arrested and 115 were merely reported by NAS to the judicial authority; no specific data about the professions of the suspects were given.) Other sources, reviewed below, provide evidence of several other investigations.

- Less surprisingly, given plausible connections to body-building, "owners or managers of a dietary supplement shop" make up the third largest category of suspects in the database. The database reports 61 such suspects in eight different investigations.
- Pharmacists constitute the fourth largest professional category in the database. In total, 20 pharmacists are suspected of doping-related violations in nine different investigations. Moreover, an unspecified number of pharmacists were reported in five other investigations.
- The database also lists 17 accommodating or corrupt physicians.

The remaining categories, in rank order, consist of staff members of cycling teams; sports federation officials; law enforcement or military officers; employees of public hospitals, including nurses; employees or representatives of pharmaceutical and dietary supplement companies; and employees of private security firms. If we were to consider team and federation affiliates as a single "organized sports" category, see below, they would rank ahead of pharmacists and physicians.

6.3 A typology of the suppliers of doping products

On the basis of the professional and occupational delineations and rankings in the NAS database and all the criminal proceedings, I have identified ten main types of illegal suppliers of doping products in Italy and grouped them in five over-arching categories (see Table 6.2).

Gym

The first category, "gym," consists of two types of illegal suppliers that are ranked highly among all professionals and occupations in the NAS Investigations Database: "gym owners or managers and body-building instructors," and "owners or managers of dietary supplement shops." These individuals work most often as retailers, selling doping products (primarily anabolic steroids but also stimulants) to gym patrons. Some of these individuals, though, are also wholesalers, selling to retailers, who are often other gym managers, instructors, or body-builders. The manager of a gym in Forlì, for example, supplied not only several visitors to his gym but also the managers of at least four other gyms with anabolic steroids and other drugs (Tribunale di Forlì, 2009: 16–19). So did the owner of a gym specializing in body-building in Naples, who also distributed steroids and other drugs through a small network of accomplices (NAS Napoli, 2003).

According to the experts interviewed, three (former) gym owners surpass all other known steroid suppliers for the length and scope of their illegal businesses.

Table 6.2 The types of suppliers of doping products in Italy

Category	*Type*
Gym	Gym managers or owners and body-building instructors Managers or owners of dietary supplement shops
Health care	Pharmacists Physicians Hospital employees Employees, sale representatives of (para-)pharmaceutical companies
(Human) organized sports world	Staff members of sports teams Staff members of sports federations
Horseracing	Veterinary physicians, breeders and drivers
Semi-professional sportspeople	Elite athletes, and their family members Hard-core body-builders, including law enforcement, military and private security company staff, and their family members
Other	People with no distinctive profession or occupation

Source: our elaboration on the basis of NAS investigations, all criminal proceedings and media sources.

The NAS described the supplier operating on the largest scale as the " 'big father' of national and international trafficking in anabolic steroids" (NAS Bologna, 2000: 233). This former employee of the Pesaro tax collection office, body-builder, and gym owner was first reported for the illegal import and distribution of anabolic steroids in 1993. His agenda referred to seven Italian pharmaceutical companies, two pharmacies, and a private hospital as likely sources, and revealed contacts with pharmaceutical companies across Europe and in Latin America and with numberous international couriers; in the late 1990s, he supplied the two other large-scale suppliers and had direct contacts with at least 27 other gyms located in more than half of Italy's 20 regions (NAS Bologna, 2000: 243–244 and 267–268). Regarding the longevity of his involvement, the so-called "big father" was arrested in 2011 in Ancona for the illegal importation of doping products. In a storehouse under his control, the NAS seized doping products valued at over one million euros, which had been produced in clandestine laboratories in Spain, the Netherlands, and the UK (Frezzi, 2011).

Health care

The second category, "health care," consists of pharmacists, physicians, hospital employees, and employees or sale representatives of pharmaceutical and para-pharmaceutical companies (including manufacturers and distributors).

Pharmacists usually work as retailers of doping products, but also occasionally as producers of other own doping substances (Tribunale di Bologna, 2004; Capodacqua, 2001) and even more rarely as wholesalers (NAS Brescia, 2011; Int-Pro-4; Ryan, 2011). They may also be involved unwittingly in the sale of performance-enhancing drugs; that is, without awareness of the illegal intentions of the purchases. Most frequently, these "non-guilty" pharmacists sell doping drugs on the basis of either false or stolen prescriptions or prescriptions written by accommodating or corrupt physicians (e.g., Tribunale di Ravenna, 2004: 122, Int-NAS-17 and 19). However, the line between the deceived and corrupt pharmacist is sometimes difficult to draw.

Several NAS investigations point to the role played by physicians in the supply of doping products, though few of these criminal proceedings ended with convictions. Here, I summarize the story of Prof. Francesco Conconi, both as a high-profile and well-documented example of a physician's involvement with doping products and to explore the chronology of doping prohibitions in sports rules and Italian law.[2]

In the late 1970s, Conconi started providing doping products to Italian elite athletes, primarily in track and field, cycling, swimming, pentathlon, rowing, and ski sports, with the tacit support of the Italian Olympic Committee (CONI; Tribunale di Ferrara, 2003; Procura della Repubblica presso il Tribunale di Ferrara, 2000), despite the fact that the IOC Medical Commission had already published a first list of prohibited substances in 1967 and introduced drugs tests at the Olympic Winter Games in Grenoble and at the Olympic Games in Mexico in 1968 (Henne, 2009).

Conconi's practices were also illegal under Italian law. With Act 1099 of 1971, athletes' use of doping substances and the administration of such substances to athletes were criminalized, albeit as a misdemeanor, not a felony (Arioli and Bellini, 2005). These offences were depenalized in 1981 and a new specific bill on doping was not adopted until 2000 (Arioli and Bellini, 2005). However, even before 2000, the administration of doping substances to elite athletes not only violated sports rules but also met the requirements of other offenses foreseen by the Italian penal code and special bills. The most relevant one is the offense of "administration of drugs in a dangerous way for public health" (article 445 of the Italian Penal Code, hereinafter CP). Another applicable offense was that of "sporting fraud," which was introduced with Act 401 of 1989. The bill was prompted by the first match-rigging scandals in football and the difficulties of applying the general offense of fraud to them (Tribunale di Bologna, 2004: 10–11). Over time, this bill was also used to prosecute crimes related to doping, albeit in a partially controversial manner (see Paoli and Donati, 2014: 153–154).

In the main trial Conconi was charged with sporting fraud (Tribunale di Ferrara, 2003). In a related proceeding, Conconi and high-ranking CONI officials were charged with criminal association for the purpose of distributing drugs in a dangerous way to public health (article 445 CP) (Procura della Repubblica presso il Tribunale di Ferrara, 2000; see section 6.5 below). In the first instance, the case was eventually dismissed because it triggered the statute of limitations;

in the second instance, the charges themselves had to be dropped for the same reason.

Until the late 1980s, Conconi's most effective application consisted of blood doping or analogous transfusions, a doping method that was allegedly also applied in those years in other countries (e.g., Finland, see Doping Enquiry Taskforce, 2001). The Italian Ministry of Health banned blood transfusions for non-therapeutic purposes in early 1986 (Donati, 2012: 46–48); the IOC followed closely on that in the same year. Even before those bans, however, analogous transfusions were not a standard therapeutic or research practice and most specialists, including Conconi himself, knew that these transfusions might de facto constitute doping.[3]

Beginning in the early 1990s, Conconi began using erythropoietin (EPO) and increasingly substituted "emo (that is, blood)-doping" with "epo-doping." Under the auspices of doping research that was funded by CONI (with sums amounting to more than two million euros over the years; see Tribunale di Ferrara, 2003), Conconi was able to achieve noteworthy results with the athletes working with him. At the 1994 Winter Olympics, Italy won 34 medals in long-distance skiing; it was later documented that many of these athletes registered hematocrit values[4] of greater than 50 percent – a strong indication of EPO use and measurements that, today, would require suspension from competition (Bellotti, 1999; Akinde, 2006).

By the early 1990s, Conconi had begun treating elite riders working in private teams, including well-known figures in Italian cycling; at the same time he was also a member of the IOC's Medical Committee and the President of the Medical Commission of the Unione Cycliste Internationale (UCI), and received large amounts of funding from the IOC – reportedly to develop an EPO test that he did not deliver. At the end of that decade, the Ferrara Prosecutor's Office indicted Conconi and two of his assistants of the crime of sporting fraud. Despite "the seriousness and convergence of all the evidence" (Tribunale di Ferrara, 2003: 46), the inefficiency of the Italy judicial system and the defendants' procedural tactics (e.g., Toti, 2003) left the Ferrara judge no other choice but to dismiss the case in 2003 due to the statute of limitations.

The most famous of Conconi's pupils is Michele Ferrari, a physician, who split from Conconi in the late 1990s and later specialized in attending to high-level riders, including the US rider Lance Armstrong. Armstrong was stripped of his seven Tour de France titles and banned for life from sanctioned Olympic sports by the US Anti-Doping Agency (USADA, 2012) in October 2012. As documented in the USADA's decision and reported by Hamilton (Hamilton and Coyle, 2012), Ferrari was the mastermind of the doping and training programs followed by Armstrong and some of his team colleagues: "Ferrari was our trainer," Hamilton recalls, "our doctor, our god … Lance mentioned Ferrari constantly, almost annoyingly so. *Michele says we should do this. Michele says we should do that*" (Hamilton and Coyle, 2012: 102; emphasis added).

Several investigations and related proceedings also document the involvement of hospital, health clinic and nursing home employees in the supply of doping products. Low-level health care employees may engage in theft, whereas private health clinics may provide illegal doping methods to elite riders (e.g., Pacifici and Donati, 2011: 45).

Employees and sales representatives of pharmaceutical and dietary supplement companies, who might work independently or on behalf of a company, can also play a part in the supply of doping products. Among such individuals, employees of drug distributors have been implicated in the diversion of legitimate drugs with potential doping effects from the storehouses or trucks of their companies – their involvement occurs through either suspicious disappearances or thefts (Int-NAS-9 and 26).

(Human) organized sports world

Staff members of sports teams and federations compose the third category, which I refer to as the "organized sports world." The large-scale raids repeatedly conducted by the NAS branch offices at several editions of the Giro d'Italia and in other circumstances, and the considerable amounts of drugs seized in some of these raids strongly suggest that cycling team staff members were not only aware and tolerant of the illegal doping practices of their athletes but were also actively involved in such practices (e.g., Int-NAS-16, NAS Firenze, 2002). These findings seem also to be applicable to other countries, as shown by the USADA's (2012) investigations against Lance Armstrong and his US team, numerous doping scandals involving teams from different countries (e.g., Dopingkommission, 2009) as well as recent academic research (Fincoeur and Paoli, 2014; Fincoeur *et al.*, 2015).

Staff members of teams outside of cycling also engage in the supply of doping products. An investigation of the Turin Judicial Police and Prosecutor's Office found widespread illegal doping practices in the football club Juventus Turin from 1994 to 1998, years in which the team won three Italian Championships, the Champions League, the Intercontinental Cup, and Italy's Cup. The related proceeding documented the abuse of a large number of drugs at Italy's leading football team, which were bought mainly by the team and administered by the sports physician and his assistants, in some cases without obtaining the informed consent of the players. Whereas the offense of "doping" was inapplicable because it was not established until 2000, the two main defendants, Giraudo and Agricola, the manager and chief sports physician of the team, were found guilty of sporting fraud by Italy's Supreme Court, Corte Suprema di Cassazione (2007), for purchasing and administering illegal performance-enhancing substances, such as corticosteroids.

The line between the staff members of sports teams and the officials of sports federations is often thin and blurred; however, it is an important analytical distinction, as the latter belong to sports ruling bodies. Several proceedings based on NAS investigations and other sources (e.g., Donati, 1989 and 2012) report the involvement of sports federation officials in doping practices, both as direct suppliers and as "protectors."

Horseracing

The fourth category refers to the world of horseracing and includes breeders, veterinarians, and drivers. I discuss these three types of suppliers jointly, as the NAS Investigations Database and other sources do not provide specific information on each. Several investigations, both in southern and northern Italy, have shown that numerous veterinary physicians, breeders and drivers exchanged doping products and administered them to horses to "fix" the results of official competitions and thus earn considerable sums of money with legal and illegal bets (e.g., Fazzo and Mensurati, 2002; *Repubblica*, 2008).

Semi-professional sportspeople

The fifth category, "semi-professional sportspeople," consists of elite athletes, hard-core body-builders, including law enforcement, military and private security company staff, and, in some instances, their family members. NAS investigations, other criminal proceedings and media reports indicate that some elite athletes and hard-core body-builders do not just use doping products to improve their own performance but they or their closest family members also engage in the import and distribution of doping substances Some of these individuals purchase doping products for their own consumption, but then sell additional amounts to others, either to finance their own consumption or to earn extra money.

Given frequent trips abroad, elite athletes may be ideally positioned to import doping substances, especially from countries, regions, or localities with less restrictive regulations or relatively lax enforcement. Exploiting differences in national, regional, or local regulations and enforcement, they also may be able to buy some of these products legally or without detection or risk of penalty and then sell the amounts in excess of their consumption needs to other people, who might be users or dealers. Most athletes who acquire doping products do so to improve their athletic performance, but a few also sell them to others (e.g., NAS Brescia, 2011).

Just as elite athletes, hard-core body-builders, too, occasionally trade in the same doping products they consume. Since the 1990s, NAS investigations and other proceedings have provided repeated evidence of body-builders operating as user-dealers and, more rarely, as wholesalers. Among them, law enforcement, military and private security company personnel compose a numerically consistent and particularly worrying subtype. Body-building is an attractive activity among police officers and private security personnel, both of which are usually associated, especially at low-levels, with an athletic and imposing physical presence (Hoberman, 2012). To the extent that body-building law enforcement and military officers or private security personnel become involved in the supply of doping projects, most of them remain user-dealers and only a few expand the scope of their businesses beyond retail (e.g., Tribunale di Bologna, 2000; Tribunale di Forlì, 2009; Numa, 2010; Tribunale di Torino, 2012).

Other illegal suppliers

The final category of illegal suppliers consists of "other" persons with none of the above-mentioned distinctive professions or occupations. Most of them also have a legitimate profession or occupation, ranging from salesman to student, but the NAS database does not enable us to quantify them. In this residual category, we also find a few suppliers active in the thoroughly illegal segments of the market for doping products, as producers of doping substances in illegal labs, thieves, truck hijackers, or operators of specialized websites. A good illustration of this type of supplier is the jobless former nurse of a Turin hospital, who produced anabolic steroids in a lab close to Brescia and marketed them through a website on behalf of an international criminal organization (Int-NAS-9).

6.4 Distribution chains and market relationships

After classifying the suppliers of doping products, Paoli and Donati (2014) identified the sources and distribution levels of the different doping products, distinguishing between doping substances and methods, on the one hand, and among different doping substances, on the other. Such an exercise also allowed them and me to establish the extent to which a "market," as defined above, exists.

In the case of doping methods, we conclude that no separate quasi-illegal market exists. Doping methods are administered on an ad hoc basis to elite athletes by a limited number of physicians and private clinics using legitimate and often banal medical instruments. Whereas there is a legitimate market for such instruments entailing multiple and competing distribution chains, there are no regular exchanges for doping methods. However, final users can, to a large extent, functionally substitute the most frequent doping method, i.e., blood transfusion, with doping substances, specifically EPO.

Given the multiple and competing distribution chains supplying the final users, there is obviously a market for doping substances in Italy – and probably elsewhere. Money, though, might not change hands in the final transactions between users and suppliers (e.g., when suppliers are team staff members). The distribution chains differ in their length depending on the substances and quantities traded and the degree of entrepreneurship of the final users, and by legal status, depending partly on some of the same factors. The legal status of the particular exchanges and transactions along a distribution chain might also vary by context. Some substances, especially steroids, are produced exclusively for doping purposes in pharmacies or in illegal labs, in Italy or abroad. A large, but not precisely known, share of the doping substances sold in Italy appears to have been produced by legitimate drug manufacturers located in Italy or abroad and to have been diverted at some stage from the legal distribution chain. As Italian anti-doping investigations indicate, the diversion can take place at different levels of the distribution chain. Employees or managers of the Italian or foreign drug manufacturers or their distributors may decide to divert some of the legal production to the illegal market. Drugs may also be stolen from storehouses or trucks of drug distributors or from hospitals or, more rarely, pharmacies by personnel of these institutions or by external thieves in Italy and abroad. Italian and foreign pharmacists may also intentionally divert doping products, but still be unaware of the non-therapeutic purposes for which some of their customers buy drugs and then sell them, either on the basis of a prescription written by a corrupt physician or of a false or stolen prescription. In some foreign (non-Italian) countries, pharmacists may be allowed, under domestic laws, to sell drugs, the sale and use of which are, however, restricted in Italy.

Given the multiplicity of doping products available in the market and the fact that, within each class of products, such as steroids or stimulants, several products can be functionally equivalent, users can engage with a variety of retailers, each representing the final link of an alternative distribution chain that might be part of a different system. Moreover, the availability of doping products has increased tremendously with the spread of websites selling steroids and other pharmaceuticals. Internet sales have made it possible for users in Italy – and elsewhere – to bypass domestic distribution chains, by ordering doping products online and having them delivered by mail at home.

Unlike illegal drug traffickers or dealers, the majority of the suppliers of doping products can hide their illegal transactions and their relationships with their "doping partners" – their own suppliers, collaborators, and customers or patients – behind the legitimate roles they play in their businesses, organizations, or professions. The embeddedness of doping-related supply-side activities in legitimate professions, roles, and institutions often makes the development of separate illegal enterprises to run these activities unnecessary. That embeddedness is also suggestive of white-collar crime (Sutherland, [1949] 1983), and the related and partially overlapping concepts of occupational, corporate (Clinard and Quinney, 1973), and organizational crime (Schrager and Short, 1978): these range from employee theft and other low-level crimes to high-level crimes and violations on behalf or against organizations (see also Braithwaite, 1985).

However, some illegal suppliers have trouble finding a professional cover to hide the production, import (i.e., smuggling), and wholesale distribution of doping products outside the regular channels or the product diversion from these channels. At the higher levels of the market, i.e., closer to the point of production, and especially for steroids, illegal enterprises sometimes develop that are similar to those operating in illegal drug markets. Like drug enterprises in developed countries (e.g., Reuter, 1983; Pearson and Hobbs, 2001; Paoli *et al.*, 2009), illegal enterprises producing doping substances at least in Italy tend to remain small and incorporate illegal relationships and transactions into blood or family relationships to reduce their vulnerability to law enforcement efforts.

Reflecting the white-collar background of many or most suppliers, the suppliers of doping products in Italy, other than truck hijackers, are rarely reported to use violence. Except for a single, poorly organized attempt, the anti-doping investigations and our respondents also provide no evidence of suppliers of doping products bribing or attempting to bribe public officials. Even if they do not resort to violence or bribes, some suppliers of doping products cheat their customers by manufacturing or selling counterfeited products – perhaps to a larger extent than their counterparts in illegal markets. Particularly in elite sports, different types of suppliers – e.g., physicians, pharmacists, coaches, and sports federation officials – also abuse their positions of authority and the athletes' and the athletes' parents' trust by prescribing, selling or administering the athletes doping products and convincing them of the necessity and harmlessness of doping products.

6.5 The role of national sports bodies

The most startling peculiarity of the elite segment of Italy's market for doping products is the once-common protection provided by officials and staff members of sports authorities, such as CONI, and key sports federations, many of whom were civil servants and some of whom even served as government representatives. In a small number of well-documented cases (see, e.g., Donati, 2012), these officials and staff members served as outright suppliers of doping products.

As the criminal proceedings indicate, the representatives of national sports bodies, including some very high-ranking officials, acted as "protectors" until the late 1990s. A fine line might separate individuals from their institutions, but a request of partial closure filed in October 2000 by the Prosecutor's Office of Ferrara (Procura della Repubblica presso il Tribunale di Ferrara, 2000) in the proceedings against Conconi provides evidence of high-ranking individual involvement to such a degree that it might be difficult to argue against institutional complicity. After reconstructing the relationships between CONI and Conconi since the late 1970s, Ferrara Prosecutor Soprani came to the conclusion that Conconi had set up a "criminal organization" (article 416 of the Italian criminal Code, CP; Procura della Repubblica presso il Tribunale di Ferrara, 2000: 42) together with three CONI Presidents – Franco Carraro (CONI President from 1981 to 1986), Arrigo Gattai (CONI President from 1987 to 1994), Mario Pescante (CONI Secretary General from 1981 to 1994 and CONI President from 1995 to 1998) – and the head of the Research and Documentation Section of the CONI School of Sport, Gianfranco Carabelli. This criminal association had allegedly the purpose of distributing drugs in a way dangerous to public health (article 445 CP) and was active throughout the 1980s, but not in the 1990s (Procura della Repubblica presso il Tribunale di Ferrara, 2000; see also Capodacqua, 2000).[5] Pescante and Conconi were regarded as the promoters of the criminal organization. Because too much time had elapsed between the alleged activities and the prosecution, Soprani was required to drop the charges but insisted that his request of closure "does not diminish the social and criminal non-value of the activities proved" (Procura della Repubblica presso il Tribunale di Ferrara, 2000: 56).

None of the four top officials of CONI who were indicted by the Ferrara Prosecutor's Office chose to appeal the prosecutor's charges and, surprisingly, at least for outside observers, the charges did not appear to negatively impact the suspects' sports or political careers. Pescante, for example, became undersecretary for sports in 2001, less than a year after the prosecutor's request was filed, and held that position until 2006. "Appointing Pescante to stand guard over sports is a bit like putting a fox in charge of the henhouse," complained the journalist Travaglio (2005). From 2004 to 2006, Pescante was also the Italian government supervisor for the 2006 Winter Games in Turin. In that capacity, Pescante repeatedly asked, at the IOC's insistence, for the temporary suspension of the Italian anti-doping law (Tropeano, 2005; Vinton, 2005). His international career does not appear to have suffered either. Pescante has been an IOC member since 1994, without interruption, and was the first Italian to become an IOC Vice-President in 2009.

The protection granted by Italian sports bodies to elite athletes and those administering doping products to them goes beyond Conconi's case. Another prominent example is the 1998 investigation that led to the temporary closure of CONI's anti-doping laboratory in Rome and the withdrawal of its IOC accreditation. Searches ordered by the Turin prosecutor, Raffaele Guariniello, demonstrated that the lab did not carry out proper tests for steroids in 70 percent of the urine samples of Italy's football league players. Positive tests were covered up and documents were destroyed (Evaluation Team, 2002: 13; and Travaglio, 1998). A commission of inquiry established by the government concluded that "the number of violations recorded in the mechanisms to ascertain prohibited substances specifically in football was so large as to compromise the whole anti-doping policy pursued by CONI" (*Adnkronos*, 1998).

Since the year 2000, no cases of overt high-level complicity have come to the fore, but the national sports bodies' apparent lack of interest in a thorough fight against doping still emerges from their actions and inactions, including the sports federations' lack of collaboration with law enforcement agencies and their record on testing (Paoli and Donati, 2014: 37, 116–119; CONI, 2012). In its turn, UNIRE, the public body in charge of regulating horseracing, was almost unanimously considered to be very corrupt and poorly managed (Zunino, 2009), so much so that it was re-founded in 2011 under a new name.[6]

Past and ongoing scandals involving top athletes and national sports federations and anti-doping agencies in other countries, such as Finland (Doping Enquiry Taskforce, 2001; Hahn and Häyrinen, 2008), Austria (IOC, 2007), the former East Germany (Berendonk, 1991; Spitzer, 2013) and West Germany (Spitzer *et al.*, 2015) and Russia (Independent Commission, 2015), as well as in key international federations such as the UCI (Cycling Independent Reform Commission, 2015) and the International Association of Athletics Federations (IAAF, Independent Commission, 2015) raise the suspicion that Italian government and sports bodies were not alone in tolerating of even actively supporting their respective elite athletes' doping practices. The East German doping program was, for example, top-down and involved practices that were found, after Germany's reunification in 1989, to amount to grievous bodily harm and led to several convictions in Berlin courts.

6.6 The role of organized crime

The analysis of the criminal proceedings and the expert interviews indicate a very limited involvement of southern Italian mafia groups in the production and distribution of doping products. Among the suppliers considered so far in this chapter, there is only one specific type that can be traced back to southern Italian mafia-type organized crime groups: the hijackers stealing doping substances from trucks, who are often associated with Neapolitan camorra groups. Members of some camorra groups also play an important role in fixing horse races, which is often achieved by doping horses. These practices lend some, albeit narrow, support to WADA's assessment that the same underworld people who trade in doping substances also undermine the integrity of sports through illegal betting.

The illicit enterprises set up by some suppliers of doping products and the looser partnerships developed by others, even within legitimate institutional contexts, meet, at least in Italy, the very loose requirements of the definitions of organized crime set forward at the international level, including that of the 2000 UN Convention against Transnational Organized Crime (UNGA, 2000). Regardless of the labels chosen, one should not forget the fact that, with the exception of a limited number of underworld characters, most suppliers of doping products are not typical organized crime or underworld figures; they have a legitimate professional background, with a non-negligible share of them belonging to the organized sports world.

6.7 A semi-illegal market

The previous analysis leads me to conceptualize the doping market as a quasi-illegal market, at least from the point of view of criminal law. The legal status of doping products suffers the burden and ambiguity of contextual specificity; that is, in some contexts, the products, including their supply, are "legal" and in others they are not. In that way they are more like diverted pharmaceutical products and less like traditional illicit substances, such as cocaine and heroin. By and large, society treats the latter as "inherently" illegal: most countries prohibit trafficking and possession of cocaine, heroin and other illegal drugs for non-personal use because, with few exceptions, these drugs have been deemed dangerous to public health and lacking therapeutic value. Instead, most doping products are also legitimate, well-established pharmaceutical products.

The legal status of many supply-side activities varies along the distribution chain. A drug may begin its "life" as a legal product at one end of the supply chain and conclude its "life" as an illegal product at the other. Many drugs which are used illegally as doping products are produced by legitimate pharmaceutical companies that may not meet the regulatory requirements of Western developed countries but can operate lawfully in their own countries.

Given the lack of harmonization of the relevant criminal law legislation on doping even within the EU, the same supplying activities are likely to have different legal statuses in different countries. Body-builders in Germany can legally obtain anabolic steroids through regular physicians and pharmacies (Striegel *et al.*, 2006), whereas physicians and pharmacists cannot legally prescribe or sell the same drugs to body-builders in Italy. In a comparative perspective it is also necessary to ascertain the effective degree of enforcement of the existing regulations and prohibitions (for the concept of "effective illegality," see Paoli, *et al.*, 2009). Numerous observers (e,g, Hoberman 2011: 100) complain that even the existing sports rules and criminal law provisions have not always been implemented effectively.

Even within the same country, some doping products, with very restricted therapeutic uses, may be "more" illegal – at least from the point of view of criminal justice rather than sports authorities – than others. Leaving aside "traditional" illegal drugs, such as cocaine and cannabis, which are also on the WADA Prohibited List, nandrolone is a good case in point. In 2010, the Italian Ministry of Health added nandrolone, an anabolic steroid, to the list of psychoactive substances to be controlled under Italian drug law (DPR 309/1990 and later amendments), therefore sharply reducing the possibility of its legal sale and consumption and allowing a whole range of special investigation methods (e.g., controlled delivery) that are not allowed by Italy's anti-doping act (Ministero della Salute, 2010).

According to Italian legislation, many actors frequently involved in the supply of doping products, such as physicians or pharmacists, may or may not commit a crime depending on the therapeutic needs of their customers and clients. Specifically, the legality or illegality of their decisions and actions depends on whether their customers and patients are athletes consuming certain products "in order to improve [their] competitive performance" (article 9 of Act No. 376/2000). At one extreme, prescribing or materially supplying a performance-enhancing product to an athlete taking part in competition always constitutes a crime according to the Italian anti-doping act. At the other extreme, supplying the same product to a patient, including an athlete, who needs it for therapeutic reasons never constitutes a crime. Between these two extremes, there is an ambiguous continuum where the legal status of the physicians' or pharmacists' decisions and actions depends on whether offenses other than those foreseen by the anti-doping act are applicable and on the physicians' assessment of patient's psycho-physical conditions and needs.

The potential applicability of multiple offenses to doping contributes to the ambiguous legal status of supply-side activities. As apparent in the short discussion of doping regulation in Italy in relation to the Conconi case and the more systematic analysis of NAS investigations and related criminal proceedings conducted elsewhere (Paoli and Donati, 2014: 179–187), the supply of doping products has been criminalized and punished in Italy with reference to various offenses, beyond that of doping.

In fully illegal markets, both parties in a transaction are usually aware of the illegal nature of the exchange, even if, as might occur in Italy, the drug user does not necessarily commit a criminal offense if buying drugs solely for personal consumption. In the case of doping, one of the parties to a transaction involving doping products may be ignorant of any illegality or rule-breaking, reflecting the "embeddedness" of doping exchanges in legitimate social networks and professional activities. This is, for example, the case of a pharmacist who sells a doping product on the basis of a fraudulent or stolen prescription.

As a result of the variable and "contestable" illegality of many doping transactions, most of the suppliers of doping products, including retailers, are very different from the stereotypes of members of criminal organizations or enterprises or undocumented migrants selling wholly illegal drugs on the street. Even the illegal suppliers of doping products singled out in the NAS investigations fall outside those stereotypes; they are mostly male, Italian citizens and, with few exceptions, rarely have criminal records. The analysis of the criminal proceedings and the expert interviews also indicate a very limited involvement of southern Italian mafia groups in the production and distribution of doping products.

The quasi-illegality of many doping exchanges also reduces the risks of many suppliers and pushes down their profit margins. As only a single illegal lab has been seized in Italy, there are few direct data to assess the profit margins of the producers of doping substances. What we do know is that at least until the advent of Internet trading, large-scale traffickers and specifically the importers (were able to) generate considerable, but not sensational, revenues. Working as consultants in a criminal investigation, Donati and Magrì (2001) estimated that two of the largest-scale suppliers of doping substances among gym patrons each raised about two billion lire (approximately one million euros) annually at the turn of the century. At year-2000 prices (UNODCCP, 2001: 213), the same sum could be generated with the sale of less than 30 kilograms of cocaine.

There are also a few people in Italy, however, who generate considerable income with doping products. These appear to consist of the physicians who "treat" super-elite athletes and a large clientele of anonymous clients with doping methods and other performance-enhancing products. According to the ongoing investigation coordinated by the Padua Prosecutor's Office, for example, Michele Ferrari earned at least several million euros annually until 2011 (Int-Pro-3; Int-NAS-10; USADA, 2012).

Many other markets are also quasi-illegal, as they involve goods and services that are not thoroughly prohibited but that can, under some conditions, be sold, bought, and used legally. Consider, for example, the differences between the "white," "grey," and "black"[7] components of the markets for cigarettes, weapons, gambling, and, most notably in the context of doping, painkillers. Notwithstanding the temptation to look to illegal drug markets – specifically, heroin and cocaine – for policy models and insight, they, as wholly illegal markets, might present weak analogies for a study of doping products. Thus, anti-doping policy-makers and researchers might be called to turn to different analogies and their related literatures to draw out the implications of variations in legality for anti-doping policy.

Notes

1 Paoli and Donati (2014) refer to these interviews with the following codes: Int-NAS-1 to 26 for the NAS officers, Int-Proc-1 to 7 for the prosecutors and Int-Oth-1 and 2 for the two others, and I use these same codes here.
2 Prof. Francesco Conconi has been a professor of biochemistry at the University of Ferrara since 1967, is the current head of its Centro di Studi Biomedici applicati allo Sport, and was Rector of the same university from 1998 to 2004. See his personal webpage at http://docente.unife.it/francesco.conconi/curr.
3 In an interview quoted in an official document of the Ferrara Prosecutor's Office, Conconi stated that analogous transfusion

> may be doping but before classifying it as such we need to analyze the reasons why the technique of analogous transfusion is carried out on an athlete. If one aims to treat a subject who has a hemoglobin level lower than average and to raise that level to the average, then an analogous transfusion performs only a therapeutic function, because it "normalizes" an anomalous situation. If instead, one deals with a subject with normal hemoglobin values and adds up blood to enhance performance, then this operation can be seen as doping.
>
> (Donati, 2012: 37–38)

4 That is, the volume percentage (%) of red blood cells in blood.
5 Employees other than the physicians who may also work in these institutions.
6 Despite "a multiplicity of circumstantial evidence" (Procura della Repubblica presso il Tribunale di Ferrara, 2000: 52), the prosecutor found, instead, no conclusive proof of the existence of a criminal organization between Conconi and the top CONI leaders after 1989.
7 The terms "white," grey," and "black" are not subject to hard-and-fast definitions, but for current purposes the following distinctions are made: "white" markets are wholly legal; "grey" markets violate terms of distribution, but neither the channels nor the products are illegal, per se; and "black" markets involve illegal trade, but not necessarily illegal products. In some cases, however, as in that of cigarettes, legality can also depend on the terms of use.

References

Adnkronos. 1998. Commissione Grosso: Doping, 'Federcalcio Corresponsabile'. Available at: www.adnkronos.com/Archivio/AdnAgenzia/1998/10/14/Sport/COMMISSIONE-GROSSO-DOPING-FEDERCALCIO-CORRESPONSABILE_172900.php.

Akinde, M. 2006. Cycling's winter of discontent. The reason why. *Daily Peloton*. Available at: www.dailypeloton.com/displayarticle.asp?pk=10163.

Arioli, G. and V. Bellini. 2005. *Disposizioni penali in materia di doping*. Milan: Giuffré.

Beckert, J. and F. Wehinger. 2013. In the shadow: Illegal markets and economic sociology. *Socio-Economic Revue*, 11(1), 5–30.

Bellotti, P. 1999. Perizia del dottor Pasquale Bellotti e del centro di ematologia dell'ospedale Careggi di Firenze.

Berendonk, B. 1991. *Doping Dokumente – von der Forschung zum Betrug*. Berlin-Heidelberg: Springer.

Braithwaite, J. 1985. White collar crime, *Annual Review of Sociology*, 11, 1–25.

Bundeskriminalamt. 2011. Operation "Sladge-Hammer" und "International Pharmaceuticals." Available at: www.bmi.gv.at/cms/BK/presse/files/2_2_2011_Operation_Sladge_Hammer_und_intern_Pharmaceuticals.pdf.

Capodacqua, E. 2000. Accuse choc da Ferrara: il Coni dietro al doping. *La Repubblica*. Available at: www.repubblica.it/online/sport/pantapro/con/con.html?ref=search.

Capodacqua, E. 2001. Processo al dr. Ferrari E si riapre il caso gH. *La Repubblica*. February 13: 54. Available at: http://ricerca.repubblica.it/repubblica/archivio/repubblica/2001/02/13/processo-al-dr-ferrari-si-riapre-il.html.

Clinard, M. and R. Quinney. 1973. *Criminal Behavior Systems: A Typology* (second edn). New York: Holt, Rinehart and Winston.

CONI (Comitato Olimpico Nazionale Italiano). 2012. Dati statistici. Available at: www.coni.it/index.php?dati_statistici.

Corte Suprema di Cassazione. 2007. Sentenza sul ricorso proposto dalla Procura Generale presso la Corte d'Appello di Torino e dal difensore dell'imputato A.G. avverso la sentenza emessa dalla Corte d'Appello della stessa città in data 14 dicembre 1985. Sentenza n. Reg. Gen. N. 19255/06.

Cycling Independent Reform Commission. 2015. Report to the President of the Union Cycliste Internationale. February. Available at: www.uci.ch/mm/Document/News/CleanSport/16/87/99/CIRCReport2015_Neutral.pdf.

Donati, A. 1989. *Campioni senza valore*. Firenze: Ponte alle Grazie.

Donati, A. 2007. *World Traffic in Doping Substances*. Available at: www.wada-ama.org/Documents/World_Anti-Doping_Program/Governments/WADA_Donati_Report_On_Trafficking_2007.pdf.

Donati, A. 2012. *Lo sport del doping. Chi lo subisce, chi lo combatte*. Torino: Edizione Gruppo Abele.

Donati, A. and L. Magrì. 2001. Stima degli importi complessivi delle cessioni. Rapporto preparato per la Procura della Repubblica presso il Tribunale di Bologna.

Doping Enquiry Taskforce. 2001. Report. May 23. Available at: www.minedu.fi/edport/sites/default/OPM/Julkaisut/2001/liitteet/opm_57_dopingen.pdf?lang=fi.

Dopingkommission. 2009. Abschlussbericht der Expertenkommission zur Aufklärung von Dopingvorwürfen gegenüber Ärtzen der Abteilung Sportmedizin des Universitätsklinikums Freiburg. Available at: www.uniklinik-freiburg.de/presse/live/abschlussbericht/Abschlussbericht.pdf.

Evaluation Team. 2002. Report of the Evaluation Team. In Council of Europe (ed.) Italy: Compliance with Commitments Project – Respect by Italy of the Anti-Doping Convention. Report by Italy and the evaluation team: 31–43. Ref. T-DO (2002) 36. Available: www.coe.int/t/dg4/sport/commitments/antidoping/T-DO_2002_36_EN_eval_Report_Commit_Italy.pdf.

Fincoeur, B. and L. Paoli. 2014. Des pratiques communautaires au marché du dopage. Evolution de la distribution des produits dopants dans le cyclisme. *Déviance et Société*, 38(1), 3–27.

Fincoeur, B., K. van de Ven, and K.J.D. Mulrooney. 2015. The symbiotic evolution of anti-doping and supply chains of doping substances: how criminal networks may benefit from anti-doping policy. *Trends in Organized Crime*. Available at SSRN: http://ssrn.com/abstract=2581555

Frezzi, T. 2011. Smantellato maxi traffico internazionale di anabolizzanti. Sessantenne anconetano in manette. *Fatto e Diritto*. Available at: www.fattodiritto.it/smantellato-maxi-traffico-internazionale-di-anabolizzanti-sessantenne-anconetano-in-manette/.

Hahn, T. and R. Häyrinen. 2008. Doping im finnischen Skisport. Die schmutzigen Neunziger. *Süddeutsche Zeitung*. June 25. Available at: www.sueddeutsche.de/sport/doping-im-finnischen-skisport-die-schmutzigen-neunziger-1.203060.

Hamilton, T. and D. Coyle. 2012. *The Secret Race: Inside the Hidden World of the Tour de France: Doping, Cover-ups, and Winning at All Costs*. London: Bantam Press.

Henne, K.E. 2009. The Origins of the International Olympic Committee Medical Commission and its technocratic regime: an historiographic investigation of anti-doping regulation and enforcement in international sport. Final Report. December 31. Available at: oc.rero.ch/lm.php?url=1000,44,38,20100301152359-AF/2009_-_The_Origins_of_the_International_Olympic_Committee_Medical_Commission_-_HENNE_K.pdf.

Hoberman, J.M. 2005. *Testosterone Dreams: Rejuvenation, Aphrodisia, Doping*. Los Angeles: University of California Press.

Hoberman, J.M. 2011. "Athletes in handcuffs?" The criminalization of doping. In Mike McNamee and Verner Møller (eds) *Doping and Anti-Doping Policy in Sport: Ethical, Legal and Social Perspectives*. London: Routledge, 99–110.

Hoberman, J.M. 2012. Doping, gambling, and the decline of the IOC, mimeo.

Houlihan, B. 2002. *Dying to Win: Doping in Sport and the Development of Anti-doping Policy*. Strasbourg: Council of Europe.

Houlihan, B. and B. García. 2012. The use of legislation in relation to controlling the production, movement, importation, distribution and supply of performance-enhancing drugs in sport (PEDS). August. Available at: www.wada-ama.org/Documents/World_Anti-Doping_Program/WADP-Legal_Library/National_Legislation/UNESCO-Legislative-Research-Report-FINAL.pdf.

Independent Commission. 2015. *The Independent Commission Report No. 1*. November 9. Available at: https://Wada-Main-Prod.S3.Amazonaws.Com/Resources/Files/Wada_Independent_Commission_Report_1_En.pdf.

IOC (International Olympic Committee). 2007. Summary of the IOC Disciplinary Commission. Recommendations Regarding the National Olympic Committee of Austria. Available at: www.olympic.org/Documents/Reports/EN/en_report_1183.pdf.

Koert, A.W.A. and R. van Kleij. 1998. *Handel in doping: Een verkennend onderzoek naar de handel in dopinggeduide middelen in Nederland*. Nieuwegein: Arko.

Kokkevi, A., A. Fotiou, A. Chileva, A. Nociar, and P. Miller. 2008. Daily exercise and anabolic steroids use in adolescents: a cross-national European study. *Substance Use and Misuse*, 43, 2053–2065.

Kraska, P., C. Bussard, and J. Brent. 2010. Trafficking in bodily perfection: examining the late-modern steroid marketplace and its criminalization. *Justice Quarterly*, 27(2), 159–185.

McCabe, S.E., K.J. Brower, B.T. West, T.F. Nelson, and H. Wechsler. 2007. Trends in nonmedical use of anabolic steroids by US college students: results from four national surveys. *Drug and Alcohol Dependence*, 90, 243–251.

Ministero della Salute. 2010. Decreto 11 giugno 2010: Aggiornamento e completamento delle Tabelle contenenti l'indicazione delle sostanze stupefacenti e psicotrope relative a composizioni medicinali, di cui al Decreto del Presidente della Repubblica 9 ottobre 1990, n, 309, e successive modificazioni ed integrazioni con l'inserimento dello steroide anabolizzante nandrolone. *Gazzetta Ufficiale*, serie generale n. 145 of June 24, 2010. Available at: www.normativasanitaria.it/jsp/dettaglio.jsp?id=34277.

Ministero della Salute and Istituto Superiore di Sanità. 2012. Reporting System Doping Antidoping 2011. Available at: www.salute.gov.it/imgs/C_17_pubblicazioni_1732_allegato.pdf.

Moore, W.H. 1974. *The Kefauver Committee and the Politics of Crime, 1950–1962*. Columbia, University of Missouri Press.

NAS Bologna, Comando Carabinieri per la tutela della salute. Nucleo Antisofisticazioni e Sanità di Bologna. 2000. Procedimento penale a carico di S.M. + altri. Atti relativi all'indagine delegata sul commercio clandestino di sostanze ormonali e a effetto anabolizzante destinate al doping umano. Informativa conclusiva. Rif. Proc. Pen. n. 1701/99–21 RGNR. June 21.

NAS Brescia. 2011. Comando Carabinieri per la tutela della salute. Nucleo Antisofisticazioni e Sanità di Brescia. Informativa finale sull'esito delle indagini effettuatenei confronti di G.N. + altri.

NAS Firenze, Comando Carabinieri per la tutela della salute. Nucleo Antisofisticazioni e Sanità di Firenze. 2002. Informativa finale sull'esito delle indagini effettuate: Operazione Quadrifoglio.

NAS Napoli, Comando Carabinieri per la tutela della salute. Nucleo Antisofisticazioni e Sanità di Napoli. 2003. *Comunicazione notizia di reato (ex art. 347 CPP)* alla Procura della Repubblica presso il Tribunale di Santa Maria Capua Vetere. Procedimento penale n. 10493/2002 RGNR.

Numa, M. 2010. Anabolizzanti, poliziotti in manette: Il traffico passava dalle loro mani: 21 agenti denunciati in tutta Italia. *La Stampa*. Available at: www3.lastampa.it/torino/sezioni/cronaca/articolo/lstp/280202/.

Pacifici, R. and A. Donati. 2011. Consulenza tecnica nel procedimento penale 5876/08 Procura della Repubblica presso il Tribunale di Mantova. Mimeo.

Paoli, L. 2012. Doping and anti-doping: neglected issues in criminology. *European Journal of Crime, Criminal Law and Criminal Justice*, 20(3), 231–238.

Paoli, L. (ed.) 2014. *Oxford Handbook of Organized Crime*. New York: Oxford University Press.

Paoli, L. and A. Donati, 2014. *The Sport Doping Market: Understanding Supply and Demand, and the Challenges of Their Control*. New York: Springer.

Paoli, L., V.A. Greenfield, and P. Reuter. 2009. *The World Heroin Market: Can Supply Be Cut?* New York: Oxford University Press.

Pearson, G. and D. Hobbs. 2001. *Middle Market Drug Distribution*. London: Home Office Research, Development and Statistics Directorate.

Pope, H.G., K.A. Phillips, and R. Olivardia. 2000. *The Adonis Complex: The Secret Crisis of Male Body Obsession*. New York: Free Press.

Procura della Repubblica presso il Tribunale di Ferrara. 2000. Richiesta di archiviazione parziale. Procedimento penale control Pescante Mario + 13 altri. N. 893/99/21 R.G. notizie di reato/Mod. 21. *Repubblica, La*. 2001. Il giudice: Guandalini cedette farmaci dopanti. April 5: 4 of Bologna section. Available at: http://ricerca.repubblica.it/repubblica/archivio/repubblica/2001/04/05/il-giudice-guandalini-cedette-farmaci-dopanti.html.

Repubblica, La. 2008. Corse truccate, cavalli dopati – Nuova tegola sull'ippica italiana. Available at: www.repubblica.it/2008/12/sezioni/sport/ippica-indagine/ippica-indagine/ippica-indagine.html?ref=search.

Reuter, P. 1983. *Disorganized Crime: The Economics of the Visible Hand*. Cambridge, MA: MIT Press.

Reuter, P. 1985. *The Organization of Illegal Markets: An Economic Analysis*. Washington, DC: National Institute of Justice.

Reuters. 2007. Pfizer to pay $35 mln in Genotropin settlements. April 2. Available at: www.reuters.com/article/2007/04/02/idUSWNAS544720070402.

Ryan, B. 2011. Italian judge set to decide if 32 named in Mantova doping investigation should go on trial. Available at: www.cyclingnews.com/news/italian-judge-set-to-decide-if-32-named-in-mantova-doping-investigation-should-go-on-trial.

Schlink, L. 2011. Mafia big threat for 2012 London Olympics. *The Telegraph*. Available at: www.dailytelegraph.com.au/sport/more-sports/mafia-big-threat-for-2012-london-olympics/story-e6frey6i-1226013990795.

Schrager, L.S. and J.F. Short. 1978. Toward a sociology of organizational crime. *Social Problems* 25(4), 407–419.

Spitzer, G. 2013. *Doping in der DDR: Ein historischer Überblick zu einer konspirativen Praxis. Genese – Verantwortung – Gefahren.* Köln: Strauss.

Spitzer, G., E. Eggers, and H.J. Schnell. 2013. *Siegen um jeden Preis – Doping in Deutschland: Geschichte, Recht, Ethik 1972–1990.* Göttingen: Werkstatt.

Striegel, H., P. Simon, S. Frisch, K. Roecker, K. Dietz, H.H. Dickhuth, and R. Ulrich. 2006. Anabolic ergogenic substance users in fitness-sports: a distinct group supported by the health care system. *Drug and Alcohol Dependen*ce, 81, 11–19.

Striegel, H., R. Ulrich, and P. Simon. 2010. randomized response estimates for doping and illicit drug use in elite athletes. *Drug and Alcohol Dependence* 106(2–3), 230–232.

Sutherland, E.H. [1949] 1983. *White-Collar Crime: The Uncut Version.* New Haven: Yale University Press.

Toti, G. 2003. Caso Conconi, indietro tutta. *Corriere della Sera.* March 26: 46. Available at: http://archiviostorico.corriere.it/2003/marzo/26/Caso_Conconi_indietro_tutta_co_0_030326239.shtml.

Travaglio, M. 1998. Provette sparite, un blitz al Coni. *La Repubblica.* August 21: 46. Available at: http://ricerca.repubblica.it/repubblica/archivio/repubblica/1998/08/21/provette-sparite-un-blitz-al-coni.html.

Travaglio, M. 2005. Viva Storace – bananas. *L'Unità.* October 6: 12. Available at: http://cerca.unita.it/ARCHIVE/xml/175000/171330.xml?key=marco+travaglio&first=1461&orderby=1.

Tribunale di Bologna. 2000. Ordinanza di custodia cautelare nei confronti di P.B. + altri.

Tribunale di Bologna. 2004. Sentenza nei confronti di Ferrari Michele + 3. October 1. No. 2997/97 R.G. notizie di reato.

Tribunale di Ferrara. 2003. Sentenza nei confronti di Conconi Francesco + altri. No. 893/99 RGNG. November 19.

Tribunale di Forlì. 2009. Ordinanza di custodia cautelare nei confronti di V.M. + altri. No. 3870/07 RGNR.

Tribunale di Ravenna, 2004. Ordinanza applicative di misure cautelari nei confronti di M.A. + 73. N. 619/2003 21 R.G.N.R.

Tribunale di Torino, 2012. Ordinanza di applicazione di misura cautelari nei confronti di V.G. + 5. N. 4654/10 RGNR. July 16.

Tropeano, L. 2005. Olimpiadi: La guerra del doping. *La Stampa.* October 18: 35.

UNGA (United Nations General Assembly). 2000. *Report of the ad hoc Committee on the Elaboration of a Convention against Transnational Organized Crime on the Work of its First to Eleventh Session.* A/55/383. 2 November. Available at: www.undcp.org/palermo/convmain.html.www.undcp.org/palermo/convmain.html.

UNODCCP (United Nations Office for Drug Control and Crime Prevention). 2001. *Global Illicit Drug Trends.* New York: United Nations.

US DEA (Drug Enforcement Administration). 2007. DEA announces largest steroid enforcement action in US History. Available at: www.justice.gov/dea/pubs/pressrel/pr092407.html.

USADA (US Anti-Doping Agency). 2012. Report on proceedings under the World Anti-Doping Code and the USADA Protocol: United States Anti-Doping Agency, claimant, v. Lance Armstrong, respondent. Reasoned decision of the United States Anti-Doping Agency on disqualification and ineligibility. Available at: http://cyclinginvestigation.usada.org/

Vinton, N. 2005. Olympics: IOC ends opposition to Italy's doping laws. *New York Times.*

October 29. Available at: http://select.nytimes.com/gst/abstract.html?res=F00C16F735 5B0C7A8EDDA90994DD404482.

WADA (World Anti-Doping Agency). 2010. Minutes of the WADA Executive Committee Meeting. November 20. Montreal. Available at: www.wada-ama.org/Documents/About_WADA/ExecutiveCommittee_Minutes/WADA_ExCo_Minutes_20Nov2010_EN.pdf.

Waddington, I. and A. Smith. 2009. *An Introduction to Drugs in Sport*. Milton Park: Routledge.

Zunino. C. 2009. Sperperi e illegalità così l' ippica italiana è diventata un debito. *La Repubblica*. November 23: 21. Available at: http://ricerca.repubblica.it/repubblica/archivio/repubblica/2009/11/23/sperperi-illegalita-cosi-ippica-italiana-diventata.html.

7 INTERPOL and the fight against performance-enhancing drugs trafficking

A singular approach led by the intelligence and profiling method

Clément de Maillard and Elena Titova

Doping is an issue which has been problematic to the world of sports for several decades. The various scandals that have struck the professional sports world since the early 1990s – Festina, Balco, Armstrong, etc. – have highlighted the fraudulent behaviour of some athletes and their staff. These activities have become increasingly sophisticated and organized, to the point of using a diverse range of products and devices intended to artificially enhance performance, for the sole purpose of getting closer to victory.

Given the apparent magnitude of this phenomenon and the pressure of international bodies, during the past 30 years many countries have chosen to adjust their legal arsenal to address these issues (UNESCO, 2005). Motivated by ethical reasons such as public health, the aspiration of countries to fight against doping has led to the criminalization of the public's response. This response takes into account the dual reality of the problem: both the professionalization of doping behaviour with the sports elite, and the also worrying – although less well known – explosion of the products available to amateur athletes through the Internet (Lood *et al.*, 2012) (Thualagant and Pfister, 2012).

Despite this, doping still remains an issue generally associated with professional sports. Revelations or suspicions related to a particular elite athlete are regularly reported by the media, yet the equally alarming issue of doping in amateur sport does not attract as much attention. While the reasons for these differences may seem obvious in view of the reputation of the individuals involved and the negative image which accompanies each of these scandals, the issue of mass doping, is a very real social issue (Australian Crime Commission, 2015).

Far away from the professional sporting community with medical facilities, constant support and advanced drugs, more and more people benefit from the Internet to access the drugs and knowledge on how to increase their physical abilities or develop muscle mass. This mass doping use poses a major public health challenge. These substances are generally manufactured in clandestine and often unsanitary conditions. Producers have little regard as to the quality of their product and the risks to their purchasers. However, regardless of the product quality, the physiological risks and risks of addiction are in some respects similar to those already highlighted for the consumption of other well-known drugs – such as cocaine or heroin.

It was in this context that, in 2009, the World Anti-Doping Agency (WADA) and INTERPOL signed a partnership agreement. INTERPOL's mandate fits within its member countries' willingness to combat doping as a criminal issue by following this dual approach of focusing both on professional sports and on the mass trafficking of doping products. However, INTERPOL does not carry out investigations itself; its role is primarily to facilitate and coordinate the work of police forces internationally, and to connect them in the fight against transnational criminal issues. Its member countries retain their full sovereignty regarding legislation, investigation and prosecution. In the fight against doping, INTERPOL's mandate is threefold. First, as an international police organization, its role is to lead the exchange of information between the different police forces. Second, INTERPOL coordinates investigations – either through major operations or through a case-by-case approach. Third, INTERPOL's mission is to help the various anti-doping actors through training, awareness, participation in certain sports events alongside the police, etc. Furthermore, its proximity to WADA offers the organization the opportunity to serve as a bridge between police and the anti-doping community (laboratories, national anti-doping agencies and sporting federations).

Today, INTERPOL remains the only international law enforcement organization with specific expertise in the fight against doping. This exclusive jurisdiction does not mean that the task is straightforward, particularly in the area of combating the mass trafficking of products in the amateur sporting world.

In this area, a new approach based on current policing strategies, and more specifically the model of intelligence-led policing (Ratcliffe, 2008), has been initiated by the INTERPOL anti-doping unit. The unit is committed to making intelligence the cornerstone of its action in the fight against trafficking of doping products. As dictated by this intelligence-led model (Marclay, Jan *et al.*, 2013), this approach was applied to deconstruct and rethink the scope of action.

The first step was to frame the subject. In the context of international police cooperation, the treatment of doping is far from uniform: it is not always subject to penal action, and even when subject to prosecution, it is not always pursued by the police. In addition, every country and every legislation addresses doping and trafficking of doping substances from a different perspective. In many respects, the question of the subject definition is very significant.

Once the scope of action was defined, the second stage was to observe and analyse the nature and the specific characteristics of the topic. Indeed, the black market of doping products has as many similarities as differences with respect to other types of trafficking. Characterizing this trafficking, and identifying these differences and singularities, constituted a prerequisite to the third and final stage of this criminal intelligence process: the definition of an action plan adapted to the specific context of drug trafficking.

Defining the subject: the need for a preliminary semantic approach

The first step when addressing the issue of trafficking of doping products is to precisely define what is meant by 'doping'. The question may seem surprising but is significant as this definition varies according to its context: sporting, medical or police (Salasuo and Piispa, 2012).

From a sports point of view, a doping product is considered as any substance ingested in order to increase artificially and by unfair means the subject's performance. These products are defined in the list updated annually by the World Anti-Doping Agency according to several categories, including products banned for professional athletes in all circumstances, and those prohibited only during sports competitions (World Anti-Doping Agency, 2014).

The majority of these products have a pharmaceutical origin (growth hormones, peptide, erythropoietin (EPO), etc.), the use of which is perfectly legal under medical supervision. But the list also includes drugs as defined by the International Narcotics Control Board (INCB) whose use are prohibited for athletes and non-athletes (cocaine, amphetamine, cannabis, MDMA, etc.).

From a policing point of view, can we consider products on this list to be doping substances? In other words, does cocaine or amphetamine trafficking fall within the jurisdiction of anti-doping because these products are on the doping list? As most of the doping substances being trafficked are medicines, should this issue be considered from the perspective of the fight against pharmaceutical crime?

All these questions reveal the complexity of addressing the issue of trafficking of doping products from a police perspective.

For the INTERPOL anti-doping unit, the issue was mainly addressed through a semantic approach. First, the anti-doping unit took into account the uniqueness of the police approach: doping substances are not prohibited and drug trafficking, even of those included on the WADA list, is not within its competence. The INTERPOL anti-doping unit has therefore sought to qualify its own field of action, with a more restrictive definition than that of the sporting community.

The criterion used by the anti-doping unit for definition is the motive for consumption. This consists of substances which, through absorption, the consumer exclusively seeks to improve their physical and athletic performance. For instance, anabolic steroids and growth hormones are specifically intended for that purpose and therefore fall within this scope. However, some stimulants such as cocaine or amphetamines – while on WADA's doping list – are rarely consumed exclusively in order to improve performance. Thus, trafficking of such substances is not considered in the context of the fight against trafficking of doping products by INTERPOL. They can be taken into consideration but under the sole condition that the drug is used in order to improve performance. This may be the case, for example, when amphetamine or cocaine is mixed in a cocktail of substances intended for amateur and professional athletes to improve their performance.

To distinguish the prism through which the problem is taken into account, INTERPOL separates these products into two categories:

- With an intentionally very generic sense, the terms 'doping substances' are used for sports; they correspond to the products listed by WADA.
- For products which fit within its definition and are more relevant to police, INTERPOL uses the terminology of performance-enhancing drugs (PED).

(See Figure 7.1.)

Addressing the motive for consumption also helps to distinguish between PED and conventional drug trafficking. In both their form and their composition, performance-enhancing drugs are pharmaceutical products; they usually resemble medical products (packaging, tablets, ampoules, vials, etc.), the active substances have a pharmaceutical origin, and products from major licensed laboratories are traded on the black market (usually because they have been diverted from the legal market). In this respect, this type of trafficking should be regarded as a particular form of pharmaceutical crime. However due to its particularity, it also justifies being categorized separately. Again the motive for consumption is the differentiating criterion. Most 'classic' medicines found on the black market – either counterfeit or diverted – are aimed at those who do not have access to health care, or for whom the purchase of authorized medicines is too expensive. Most of the illegal trafficking of pharmaceutical drugs is dedicated to developing countries. However, PED are not destined for the same type of customer.

Indeed, PED consumption is mainly concentrated in developed countries. Whereas some individuals are using these for medicinal purposes, others only want to improve their image or their performance.

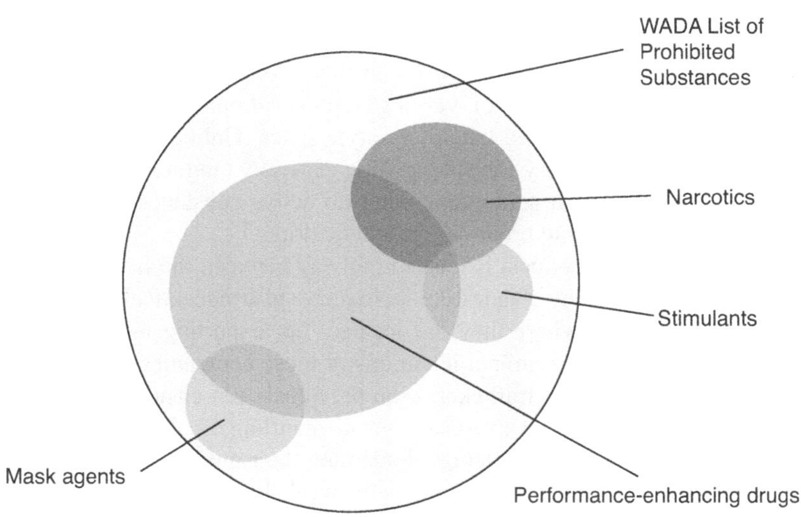

Figure 7.1 INTERPOL's definition of performance-enhancing drugs and the WADA Prohibited List.

The specific typology of the illegal market of performance-enhancing drugs justifies it being considered separately: it is neither drug trafficking nor simply pharmaceutical product trafficking. And it is precisely this typological specificity that the INTERPOL anti-doping unit aims to highlight, by analysing its characteristics including routes, actors, procedures, strengths and weaknesses. This second observation and analysis step is inscribed in the overall process of criminal intelligence implemented by the anti-doping unit whose purpose remains to define the best strategy for the circumstances.

Monitoring the environment: analysis of the PED black market and trafficking

Based on the redefinition of its scope of action and combining both its own and partners' experience, the anti-doping unit sought to highlight the typology of illegal trafficking of performance-enhancing substances by considering supply on the one hand, and demand on the other.

At the very base is the diversity of the supply chain. The PED black market is supplied in three distinct ways, each of which corresponds to different types of product. The first type are those manufactured by licensed pharmaceutical companies to treat specific diseases but diverted from the legal market. Throughout the production process, special attention has been paid to hygiene, quality and dosage. These products arrive on the black market after being diverted either directly from laboratories' stocks (which is becoming increasingly rare because of security measures), from care centres (hospitals, clinics, etc.) or from pharmacies, or were purchased legally with false medical prescriptions to be subsequently resold. Licensed products are quite rare on the PED black market, but they are also the most desirable – and therefore the most expensive – because of their reliable high quality.

The second type of product stems from an illegal origin. There are a multitude of clandestine laboratories of varying sophistication: from a converted garage to a specifically equipped laboratory-style space. Unlike licensed drugs, clandestine products are of very variable quality, generally ranging from medium to particularly harmful, with some containing no active substance at all. Such labs are similar to those found producing synthetic drugs.

The third category of products is located halfway between the licensed pharmaceutical company and the clandestine laboratory: pharmaceutical companies registered in the country where they are located, but exporting their products without a legal license. The criminal intentions of these companies are obvious: most of them were created by traffickers who previously ran clandestine laboratories. Indeed, having witnessed arrests and the dismantling of laboratories, some traffickers have realized the importance of adapting their modus operandi. They have moved their operations to countries with weak legislation, repeating the same operations but through legal companies. These people have adapted their drug trafficking to those of business leaders, but their activities have nevertheless remained the same. Their pharmaceutical companies only produce performance-enhancing drugs that are not intended for the local market but for the international market where they have no authorization to operate. Their websites – with descriptions of the discretion of shipments, the delivery confidentiality and sometimes tricks to avoid customs controls – are all evidence of their real intentions.

The question for consumers (and police) is to determine where the products they receive have come from. Given the opacity of trafficking, it is often difficult to know whether it is a clandestine laboratory or an unlicensed laboratory.

This is further complicated by another aspect that must be taken into account: counterfeiting. Indeed, some producers copy licensed brands. The irony is that even clandestine laboratories enfringe them: when a laboratory has been extremely successful on the black market other clandestine laboratories will imitate its packaging and sell their goods as such, but often with a more mediocre level of quality, to the point where it is no longer possible to distinguish the original from the copy.

And it is precisely this opacity which influences supply and demand behaviour on the PED black market. The consumer has no idea as to the origin of the products they are buying (usually on the Internet); they do not know the quality of the product purchased without a medical prescription, and have no way to assess the potential medical hazards. In this context, where information is neither pure nor perfect, the consumer will therefore seek to optimize consumption in a cost/efficiency/quality ratio. Thus, the consumer trusts a product they, or a friend, have already tested which appears effective. Discussions exchanged between consumers through online fora constantly revolve around the quality and effectiveness of a particular product or laboratory, and whether it is an original or a counterfeit.

The producer is aware of these issues, and adapts its products to coincide with consumer behaviour. Manufacturers and distributors mimic the legal pharmaceutical market by adopting codes that are supposed to give it legitimacy in the eyes of the consumer. They use a brand name and an easily identifiable logo, they play on a package's appearance to fit with traditional pharmaceutical standards by using labels, batch numbers, security codes, sometimes holograms, they have their own website and also advertise on suppliers' websites or fora. All these operations have just one goal: to reassure the potential client about the reliability of their product in order to gain loyalty.

At the same time, the efforts put into creating an attractive product exist within an environment that is opaque by nature, and therefore remain a useful source of information.

Determining the appropriate strategy: an approach to criminal intelligence

While observations of the environment including consumer habits and supply and demand behaviour provide a solid and necessary foundation of understanding, these also reveal little about key actors – suppliers or producers – of the

PED black market. Who are they, where do they come from, to whom do they sell, and how?

Given this, the INTERPOL anti-doping unit focuses only on elements that are visible to outside observers (the products themselves) and by adopting an intelligence-led approach.

Criminal intelligence uses the methodology of intelligence specifically dedicated to the fight against crime. This methodology can be illustrated as a cycle (see Figure 7.2). It encourages not only a case-by-case approach with iterative and reactive responses as dictated by each police operation, but also systematic and macroscopic processes. All newly collected material becomes part of a mosaic that this methodology aims to build in order to provide a detailed image of the phenomenon being observed. This intelligence-led approach, which emerged from police and law enforcement, has now extended to many other related components, such as forensics (Ribaux, 2014). Encouraged by some researchers and the World Anti-Doping Agency, it is also being adopted by the anti-doping community (Marclay, Mangin *et al.*, 2013).

Following this cycle, raw data is collected in accordance with the needs, and then stored according to a standardized methodology to highlight certain

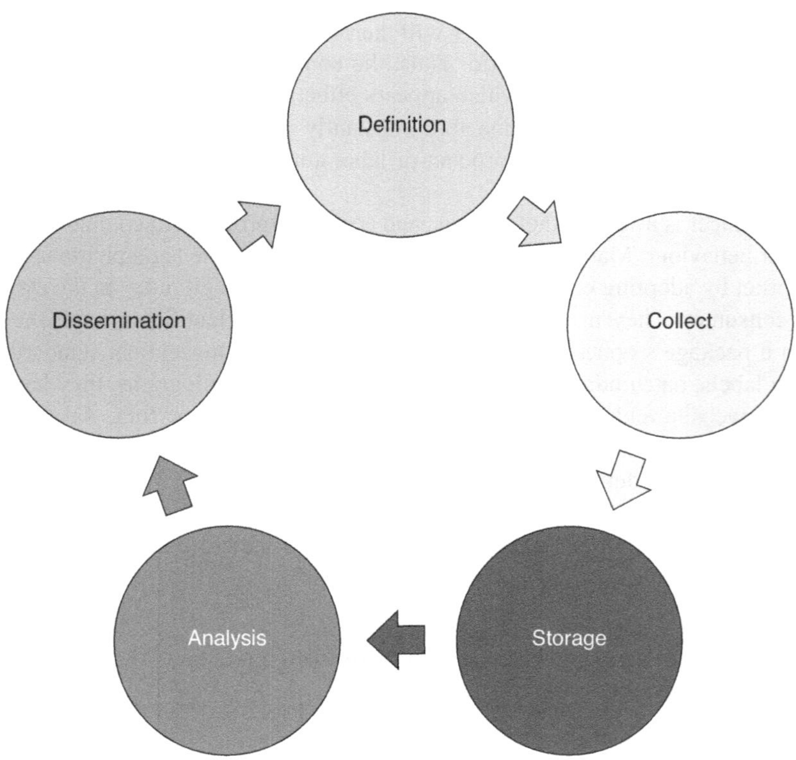

Figure 7.2 The intelligence cycle.

characteristics. Thus, from raw data these characteristics become information which, when linked and analysed, offers a different and more complete reading that can identify new perspectives.

The profiling method is a type of intelligence method: it turns raw data into information and finally into intelligence through a specifically designed intelligence cycle. Profiling consists of identifying the physical features of a product that are sufficiently unique to distinguish it from other products, and to enable comparisons with other similar types of product. The profiling method has been promoted by the academic science community (Terrettaz-Zufferey, 2009) and already implemented by various law enforcement agencies that work on narcotics (AMERIPOL, 2013; Morelato *et al.*, 2013).

Physical profiling of drugs consists of identifying the physical features of the product: logos affixed to the drug itself either by producers or their direct customers (wholesalers) to mark and identify their merchandise. But the physical profiling only remains meaningful if coupled with chemical profiling.

The chemical profiling consists of the same methodology – finding differences and potential similarities – but instead applied to the product's chemical composition. This requires determining its chemical signature: its active substance(s), features, purity and the presence of cutting products (Zadbuke *et al.*, 2012), etc. The combination of physical and chemical profiling allows for the association of the physical features of a product with its actual composition. Insofar as it may be counterfeit, the chemical analysis of the product remains the only sure method of determining its authenticity. This chemical analysis, performed with a spectrograph, reveals active substance(s) and sometimes the concentration and level of purity.

Inspired by university forensic research and the relevant experience of some pharmaceutical companies in the fight against counterfeiting, the INTERPOL anti-doping unit has recently adopted this profiling approach specifically dedicated to PED. Here, the physical profiling is based on a study of the primary packaging (to resume pharmaceutical terminology; Zadbuke *et al.*, 2012), such as the product box, and secondary packaging, containing the substance itself (vial, ampoule, blister pack, etc.). Each of these types of packaging contain a multitude of particularly useful data, such as:

- name of the PED brand mark
- active substance(s)
- information on the producer or supplier (name, contact details)
- packaging language
- batch number
- date of production
- date of expiry
- dosage.

All features identified from the analysis of primary and secondary packaging are then associated with the chemical composition of the seized product. This information is more difficult to obtain, either because many countries do not analyse the goods seized or because the results arrive later and are not subsequently forwarded to the anti-doping unit.

The profiling method is applied to all PED seized by law enforcement from INTERPOL member countries and transmitted to INTERPOL's General Secretariat. Each time a seizure of PED is reported, the anti-doping unit requests details on the products themselves. Most of the required data are defined in three categories:

- physical characteristics
- chemical characteristics
- circumstances of the seizure.

The first two categories correspond precisely to the data necessary for the profiling method. The third category, 'the circumstances', enables the contextualization of the raw data. Is it an unexpected customs seizure or a police major investigation? Who are the people involved? What is their level of involvement? What have they revealed regarding the criminal network they are involved in? What is the original country of the product? Is the country where the product was seized the final destination or a transit country? Was the product sent by mail or transported by a courier and by what method? Has a particular modus operandi been detected? Etc.

Therefore the strategy set up by the INTERPOL anti-doping unit is to ask member countries to transmit their data linked to PED seizures following predefined standards including a picture of the product, (Figure 7.3) and a systematic and continuous process. All these data are examined in detail and then stored and compared with those already collected.

This work has two types of objective: operational and strategic.

The operational side is intended to directly support law enforcement agencies in their investigations (Jan *et al.*, 2011). PED profiling provides an overview of seizures (see Figure 7.4), reveals the emergence of modus operandi, trends and recurrences, and also identifies new and unusual phenomena that deserve special attention. When such a mode of concealment is discovered, the information may be the subject of an INTERPOL Purple Notice[1] and thus be transmitted simultaneously in the four official languages of the organization to all 190 INTERPOL member countries.

The operational approach is also particularly appropriate for investigations that aim to dismantle a clandestine laboratory or a supply network (Jan *et al.*, 2011; Harcourt *et al.*, 2014). The systematic use of INTERPOL remains an asset for the country that initiates this type of investigation at a number of levels. It helps avoid duplication of effort where a various law enforcement agencies may be investigating the same protagonists (see Figure 7.5). Lack of coordination, especially internationally, can be detrimental to a favourable outcome. Good coordination specifically offers the opportunity to join forces and combine evidence. Prior to the launch of an investigation, a police department can ask whether INTERPOL has knowledge of a particular laboratory and, based on the items

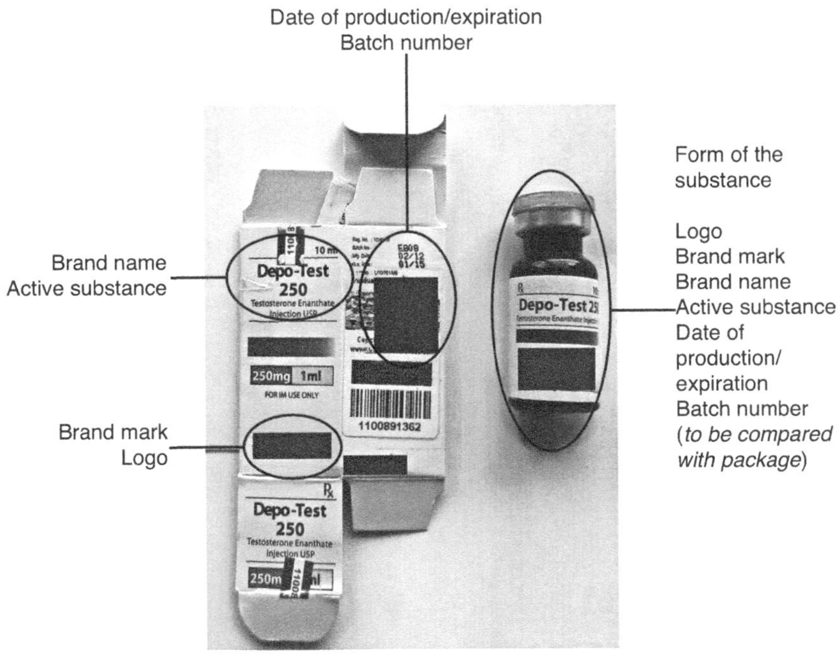

Figure 7.3 Model provided to law enforcement as a reference standard for the transmission of information related to seizures.

already registered, identify its geographical involvement (mapping), the types of products it manufactures, links with other laboratories or whether it is the victim of a copycat laboratory, etc.

Product profiling also allows elements to be linked, which when taken separately have no meaning but together highlight significant characteristics and patterns. The example of Figure 7.6 illustrates three different cases:

- In the first case, two packages found in two different seizures (seizure A and seizure B) are similar but do not have the same chemical signature. It may be a counterfeit in one of the two cases (at least), or a change in the manufacturing process.
- In the second case, the same product is seized in two different circumstances. The linkage of the two types of information gathered in both cases will feed general knowledge related to this product and distribution networks used by the manufacturer.
- In the third case, in two separate seizures, two products with different appearances prove to have the same chemical signature. This case raises the possibility of a single laboratory behind the production of these two products, even if they have two different brand marks.

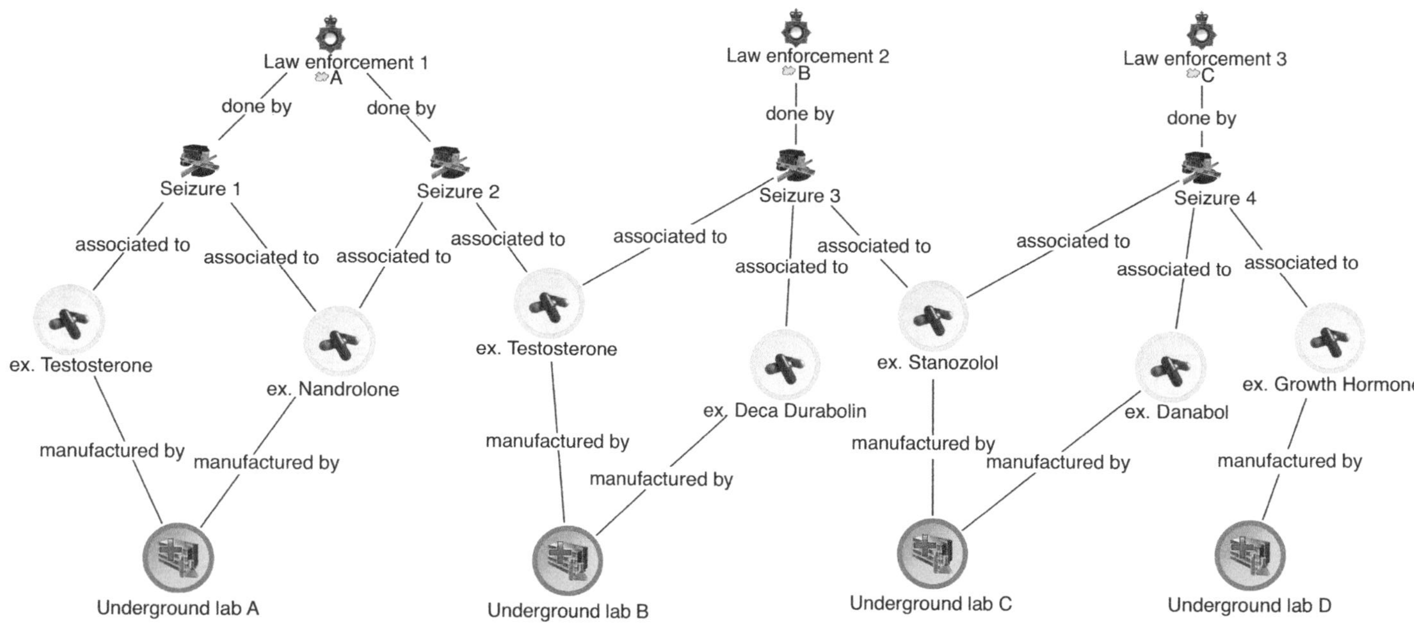

Figure 7.4 Illustration of the links between laboratories, product seizures and law enforcement agencies.

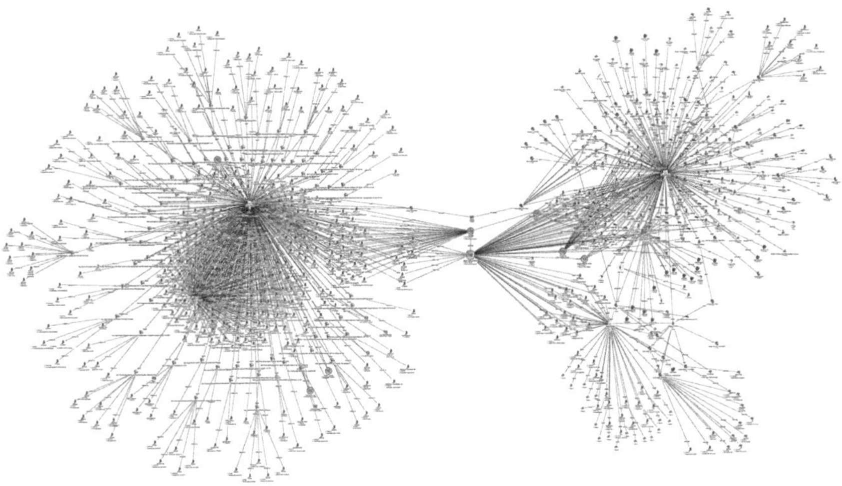

Figure 7.5 Example of links between two separate investigations related to the same clandestine laboratory.

Besides this operational analysis that supports daily police work, PED profiling also allows for strategic analysis. Strategic analysis is specifically designed to provide a global overview and improve the understanding of the phenomenon as a whole. Because it is rarer and more valuable, it is also more difficult to provide: the strategic approach stacks all of the gathered evidence piece by piece in order to determine the major trends from a quantitative point of view with statistics, or from a qualitative point of view in using observations and knowledge acquired. This analysis can be:

- about the seizures themselves: types of seizures (customs or police), performed in the framework of a delivery control or of an investigation, the countries at the origin of the largest number of seizures, those that capture the largest amounts, etc.;
- about routes and areas: production areas, transit areas, consumption areas, the main routes, methods, etc.;
- about products: the most frequent active substances or brand marks seized, cumulative quantities, trends regarding consumption, counterfeits, etc.;
- about laboratories: the most active laboratories, the links between laboratories (competition, secret links), those recently dismantled, resurgences, etc.

The main advantage of strategic analysis remains its specific ability to put all these different types of information into perspective with one another (routes and areas of a specific product, or seizures related to a specific laboratory) and highlight useful features in identifying the threat. But before being truly relevant,

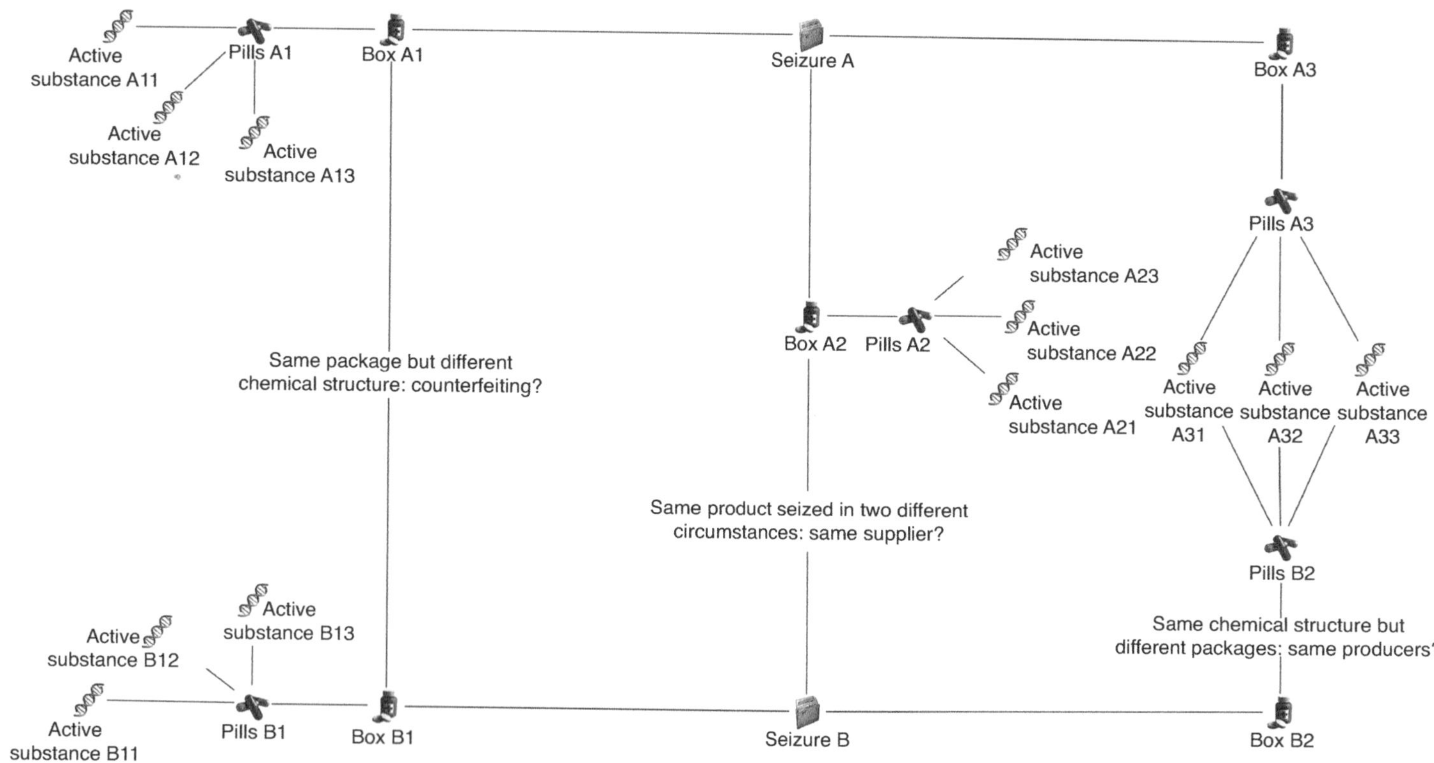

Figure 7.6 Example of different types of link highlighted by the profiling method.

strategic analysis requires the collection of a huge amount of data. At this point, the anti-doping unit does not yet have such a strategic capacity and strives to soon be able to produce such an analysis.

Performance-enhancing drugs profiling, especially its operational dimension, remains a useful and innovative initiative at the international level. Although recently established, this new initiative has already demonstrated its value.

Implementing the method: the example of 2,4-dinitrophenol case

In early 2015, after being informed of the new INTERPOL initiative, the World Anti-Doping Agency sent the anti-doping unit information obtained from the Australian anti-doping laboratory. The Australian laboratory, which works in liaison with Australian Customs, had been requested to analyse an unidentified substance of a yellow powdery appearance. The product was found to be 2,4-dinitrophenol (DNP).

DNP is a particularly dangerous substance that is mainly used as raw material in fertilizers and in the composition of some explosives. In the 1930s, it was used to increase metabolism and promote weight loss, but was quickly withdrawn as, although results were impressive, many patients died after ingesting the product. In the 1980s, medical teams attempted to reintroduce DNP as a dietary supplement. It was again removed following a patient's death, and the doctor in charge was convicted. Its ability to melt body fat quickly and effortlessly makes DNP very popular in the world of bodybuilding. Consumer fora are full of discussions on the subject with most regular users of performance-enhancing drugs reluctant to use DNP because of its bad reputation. However, if these 'regular' consumers know where they stand, other, less knowledgeable consumers are turning to DNP which is being sold as a 'magic formula' to try to resolve their obesity problems. And although the danger for these people is mainly based on lack of information related to the intrinsic dangers of the product, consumers are also unaware that the clandestine laboratories involved are not proficient in the manufacturing processes. Most of the recent deaths related to the consumption of DNP are due to an overdose of the active substance in the pill. Poorly informed consumers think that they are respecting the indicated dosage and unknowingly ingest lethal doses.

With this information, the anti-doping unit established a monitoring process in relation to DNP. One month later, in the framework of the constant contact maintained with its main partners, the anti-doping team was informed by the French Central Office for the fight against environmental damage and public health (OCLAESP[2]) that a young French man had become seriously ill a few months earlier after using DNP. In that case, the DNP had been ordered over the Internet and sent by post to the consumer's address. The following information was printed on the primary packaging:

> Health and Beauty Turmeric capsules Extra Strength 125 mg each capsule. Contains 125 mg of Turmeric Powder DO NOT USE IF SEAL IS BROKEN.

In order to divert the attention of law enforcement agents, the DNP distributors take advantage of the product's yellow powdery appearance which resembles a spice to falsely claim that the capsules contained turmeric.

These two pieces of information appeared to confirm the resurgence of 2,4-DNP on the black market or at least provide sufficient proof for it to be considered as part of investigations. With the cooperation of OCLAESP, an Orange Notice was published on 24 April 2015 to inform all INTERPOL member countries of the imminent threat posed by this substance and its resurgence on the black market. The Orange Notice was also published on the public website of INTERPOL.[3]

In the process, the INTERPOL General Secretariat issued a press release in coordination with WADA and OCLAESP. While the Orange Notice is mainly intended to inform law enforcement of the dangers of DNP and the disguised turmeric material, the press release was aimed at alerting the entire community, such as medical and health authorities, anti-doping organizations and the sporting world, but, most importantly, current and potential consumers. This global warning was coupled with a formal request for information sent to all member countries to identify and dismantle the criminal networks operating in the production and distribution of DNP. The substance 2,4-dinitrophenol is still of interest to the law enforcement community with every significant element collected, analysed and shared.

Conclusion

Today, only a few types of criminal trafficking have no international dimension. However, PED trafficking differs from other forms of trafficking – especially narcotics – by the short 'distance', logistical rather than geographical, between the producer and the consumer.

Traditional narcotics trafficking in substances such as cocaine, heroin or cannabis is generally characterized by a long supply chain. Between the producer in Latin America, Central Asia, Africa or the Middle East and the consumer in Europe or North America, for example, a considerable number of actors make up this supply chain including producers, couriers, wholesalers, semi-wholesalers, local drug retail networks, etc. In this chain, the product is cut, packaged, sold in smaller units, recut, repackaged and so on, until finally passing from the hands of a small street dealer to those of his client.

Today, the Internet is revolutionizing the PED market, becoming a significant vector for traffickers' covert activities, and there are many consequences to this change. The first of these consequences is related to the typology of the traffic. While some 'traditional' PED distribution networks[4] (running like other narcotics networks) still persist, they are now widely challenged by the Internet that offers a direct interface between supply and demand. They do not have the same structure as organized and armed territorial gangs, but rather provide flexible and opportunistic virtual networks. The virtual suppliers (on the Internet) have taken over as the actual distributors. Today, as sophisticated as they are, the links between the producer and the consumer remain much less long and complex – the products are shipped directly by couriers – and involve a much smaller number of players.

The second consequence is measured on the scale of police cooperation. While the criminal networks know how to use the Internet to expand their 'business' opportunities, they also know how to use borders to protect their activities from the police and judicial threat. Perfectly aware of the issues, they benefit from both weak or conciliatory legislation and a lack of police expertise in doping investigations in certain countries. This short 'distance' between the producer and the consumer can be problematic. The police forces with jurisdiction in the area of the PED final recipients can only try to limit the importation of the products, stopping only some consumers/retailers when legislation allows for it, while observing the biggest part of the network comfortably entrenched overseas.

The determination to fight against this trafficking, however, does not resolve this issue. The specific typology of PED trafficking on the one hand and the international dimension on the other make it necessary to rethink the approach. There needs to be a top-down approach for better harmonization of domestic legislations, combined with a bottom-up approach that focuses both on educating consumers about the dangers of trafficking and on promoting international cooperation. As only a transverse approach can be effective, these are all important parts of the fight that INTERPOL shares with its partners – in both the anti-doping and police communities.

Notes

1 INTERPOL Notices are international requests for cooperation or alerts allowing police in member countries to share critical crime-related information. There are eight types of INTERPOL Notice: red, blue, yellow, orange, green, purple, black and INTERPOL – United Nations Security Council Special Notice. Notices are published by INTERPOL's General Secretariat at the request of National Central Bureaux (NCBs) and authorized entities, and can be published in any of the Organization's official languages (Arabic, English, French and Spanish).

2 Office central de lutte contre les atteintes à l'environnement et à la santé publique.

3 The Orange Notice is still consultable online: www.interpol.int/fr/INTERPOL-expertise/Notices/Orange-notices-public-versions.

4 Outlaw moto gangs are still involved in steroids trafficking, especially in Australia (Australian Crime Commission, 2015).

Bibliography

AMERIPOL. (2013). *Catalogo de logotipos de Cocaina.* Bogota: Imprenta Nacional de Columbia.

Australian Crime Commission. (2015). *Organised Crime in Australia 2015.* Canberra: Commonwealth of Australia 2015.

Harcourt, P.R., Marclay, F. and Clothier, B. (18 March 2014). A forensic perspective of the AFL investigation into peptides: an antidoping investigation case study. *British Journal of Sports Medicine. Online First.*

Jan, N., Marclay, F., Schmutz, N., Smith, M., Lacoste, A., Castella, V. and Mangin, P. (10 August 2011). Use of forensic investigations in anti-doping. *Forensic Science International*, 213 (1–3), pp. 109–113.

Lood, Y., Eklund, A., Garle, M. and Ahlner, J. (21 May 2012). Anabolic androgenic steroids in police cases in Sweden 1999–2009. *Forensic Science International*, 219 (1–3), pp. 199–204.

Marclay, F., Jan, N., Esseiva, P., Mangin, P. and Saugy, M. (April 2013). Le changement de paradigme du Renseignement Forensique pour la lutte contre le dopage organisé et le trafic de substances interdites. *Revue internationale de criminologie et de police technique et scientifique*, pp. 451–472.

Marclay, F., Mangin, P., Margot, P. and Saugy, M. (31 January 2013). Perspectives for forensic intelligence in anti-doping: thinking outside of the box. *Forensic Science International*, 229 (1–3), pp. 133–144.

Morelato, M., Beavis, A., Tahtouh, M., Ribaux, O., Kirkbride, P. and Roux, C. (2013). The use of forensic case data in intelligence-led policing: the example of drug profiling. *Forensic Science International*, 226, pp. 1–9.

Ratcliffe, J. (2008). *Intelligence-Led Policing.* Cullompton: Willan Publishing.

Ribaux, O. (2014). *Police scientifique, le renseignement par la trace.* Lausanne: Presses polytechniques et universitaires romandes.

Salasuo, M. and Piispa, M. (2012). *Perspectives to Doping Substance Use Outside Elite Sports in Finland.* Helsinki: Finnish Youth Research Network and Finnish Youth Research Society.

Terrettaz-Zufferey, A.-L. (2009). Intégration de méthodes de data mining dans le renseignement criminel. Analyse par des structures issues de la théorie des graphes dans le profilage des stupéfiants. Doctoral thesis, University of Lausanne.

Thualagant, N. and Pfister, G. (August 2012). The fight against fitness doping in sports clubs – political discourses and strategies in Denmark. *Performance Enhancement & Health*, 1, pp. 86–93.

UNESCO. (2005). *International Convention against Doping in Sport.* Paris: UNESCO.

World Anti-Doping Agency. (2014). *The 2015 Prohibited List, International Standard.* Montreal: WADA.

Zadbuke, N., Shahi, S., Gulecha, B., Padalkar, A. and Thube, M. (2012). *Recent Trends and Future of Pharmaceutical Packaging Technology.* Maharashtra: Department of Pharmaceutics, Government College of Pharmacy, Aurangabad India.

8 Anti-doping, performance enhancement and 'the spirit of sport'

A philosophical and ethical critique

Sigmund Loland and Michael J. McNamee

Introduction

Concerns over the use of what are considered unacceptable substances and methods to enhance athletic performance are by no means new. Gleaves and Llewellyn (2014) trace the cultural roots of anti-doping to early twentieth century debates over amateurism. The anti-doping campaign gained momentum in 1967 when the International Olympic Committee (IOC) established a Medical Code with a strong message against the use of performance-enhancing drugs. Still, over the ensuing decades use of banned substances and methods among athletes has become ever more sophisticated. From the early use of androgenic anabolic steroids to increase muscle mass to micro dosing with hormones, anti-doping organizations have attempted to meet the challenges with increasing the quality of prevention, detection, and deterrence policies.

With the 1999 establishment of the World Anti-doping Agency (WADA) the anti-doping movement took a significant step forward. Co-funded by the IOC and significant sporting nation states WADA is an independent body with global authority in anti-doping. Largely through the development of its principal policy tool, the World Anti-doping Code (WADC), which is now in its third version, WADA attempts to bring greater harmonization to anti-doping work worldwide. This harmonization relates not only to testing controls and protocols, but also the developments of intelligent systems that permit location, identification and monitoring of defined groups of elite athletes with respect to the maintenance of a doping-free environment.

In addition to the scientific and medical developments, WADA has also been responsible for educational initiatives. This is a critically important aspect of anti-doping work. Success in high-performance sport has the potential of significant pay-off in terms of prestige and profit. The quest for exclusive advantages is strong. There will always be some athletes and some support systems that are willing to extend their efforts above and beyond the limits of the rules (Green, 2009). Testing control work has been largely reactive. Education aims at prevention, effectively promoting reasoned bases for why sports organizations, athletes and their support systems should commit themselves to doping-free sport. For 'education' to be worthy of that name it should have a reasoned and ethical basis. The object of this essay is to consider the ethical aspects that underpin the justification of WADA's anti-doping efforts. In order to do so, we critically consider the criteria by which substances and methods may be prohibited, and offer a more detailed ethical and philosophical interpretation of the ideal of 'the spirit of sport' than that stated in the WADC.

More specifically, we examine two main interpretations of 'the spirit of sport'. One interpretation, the 'permissive' view, builds on a view of athletes as having the freedom of choice of performance-enhancing means and methods, and of sport as an open sphere of human enhancement. An alternative interpretation, a 'restrictive' view, sees sport as a virtuous quest for human excellence. This view embraces the idea that there are clear limits to the means and methods used to enhance sporting performance. We acknowledge the seriousness and depth of some of the arguments of the permissive approach. We conclude, however, that in the current situation a restrictive view based on arguments from human excellence seems to be supported by superior reasoned argument.

Doping, facts, and values

The WADC consists of detailed regulations on the organization and carrying out of anti-doping activities. The Code is widely accepted in the scientific and sporting community. Engaging a large number of stakeholders in doping-free sport such as athletes, sports organizations, public authorities, scholars, and scientists, WADA embarked on an extensive programme of consultation in order to arrive at a policy that had greater democratic input and thus greater legitimacy than its previous counterparts. This is not to suggest that all stakeholders are committed to the WADC without criticisms or complaints, but merely to acknowledge that there has been a move away from a more paternalistic paradigm into a more consensus-driven approach.

In its more principled parts, the Code defines the concept of doping and aims at providing a justification of anti-doping. It is noteworthy how little these aspects have changed since the 1967 IOC Medical Code. In Code article 4.3, three potential criteria are set out as follows:

> A substance or method *shall be considered for inclusion* on the Prohibited List if WADA, in its sole discretion, determines that the substance or method meets any two of the following three criteria:
>
> - Medical or other scientific evidence, pharmacological effect or experience that the substance or method, alone or in combination with other substances or methods, has the *potential* to enhance or enhances sport performance.
> - Medical or other scientific evidence, pharmacological effect or experience that the use of the substance or method represents an actual or *potential* health risk to the athlete.

- WADA's determination that the use of the substance or method violates the spirit of sport described in the introduction to the Code.[1]

(Emphasis added)

The apparent simplicity of this process is deceptive (McNamee, 2012). Several important clarifications must be made before the criteria can be substantively examined. First, the criteria are those that assist WADA – specifically its Prohibited List committee – in determining whether a substance or method may be permitted or prohibited. A less noted function of this consideration may fall short of prohibition and hold that WADA will simply keep under observation the substance or method until such time as more is known about it and its effects. So the fact that a substance or method meets (at least) two of the three criteria is necessary for it to be prohibited but it is not *in and of itself* sufficient.

Second, the 'at least two from three' procedure is itself predicated on sophisticated scholarship in the philosophy of language and of law (McNamee, 2012). A complex deconstruction of this history is not relevant here. Nevertheless, it can be summarized as follows: doping in sport is a heterogeneous phenomenon ranging from the use of biochemically simple drugs for muscle growth, to exceptionally complex genetic modifications, and also to the evasion of testing control officers, or the use of other substances to mask doping substances or methods, and even extends to association with known doping personnel. In short, there are nine different offences that are collectively known as Anti-doping Rule Violations (ADRVs). The range of criteria, and the 'at least two from three' procedure, allows ADOs full scope to capture anti-doping behaviours, extending beyond the mere ingestion of banned substances, which is the commonsense – though too narrow – understanding of 'doping'. It is more precise and less open to contestation to retain the official language of the WADC and to refer to the various offences as ADRVs.

Third, even if the two first criteria are factual matters to be settled by scientific examination, applying the criteria in practice is challenging. It will be clear that the word 'potential' used in the first two criteria is open to contestation. What latitude does this open up? How likely is the actualization of harm or enhancement for it to be considered sufficient? Moreover there are other questions of a philosophical kind: what constitutes 'health risk' or what kinds or levels of health risks is anti-doping policy set against? Nor is it clear what kind of performance enhancement or what levels should trigger the concern of anti-doping policy or personnel. For example, hard training enhances performance and can also represent a risk to athlete health. Still, to most people hard training and the challenge of balancing on the right side of the catabolic and anabolic processes of the body seems to be an integrated and natural part of the challenges of sport (Loland, 2009a).

In other words, even if the extent to which a substance or method is potentially performance-enhancing and/or represents health risks to the athlete can be examined scientifically and given an evidence-based response, this is not a sufficient response to the complex of questions raised by the phenomenon of doping.

These are matters of considered judgement that require philosophical examination and clarity rather than intuitive understanding or consensus. It is noteworthy that the Prohibited List Committee does not include philosophers among its membership. Yet to precisely distinguish between acceptable and non-acceptable substances and methods, and normative premises about the nature and value of sport, is a difficult but unavoidable philosophical task. At its core, the doping debate is about ethical values. Standpoints towards doping are necessarily moral standpoints. WADA acknowledges this fact in its third criterion on the violation of 'the spirit of sport'. What are the values involved? How is 'the spirit of sport' to be interpreted?

'The spirit of sport' as a liberal view of human enhancement: a permissive account

In ethical and political terms, liberals value – perhaps more than anything else – the independence of individuals to determine the shape of their own lives. Following the classic tradition of liberalism first set out by the English philosopher and reformer John Stuart Mill (1859) in the nineteenth century, liberals believe that individuals should have autonomy and be free to determine what is in their best interests according to the shape of the life they wish to lead and consider best for themselves. They hold that society goes best when individuals are permitted this freedom. In Western democracies at least, this freedom is the subject of legal and moral rights. Nevertheless, rights to preserve and promote this freedom are not absolute. Liberals accept that there are populations, typically the young and those with impaired judgement, who are vulnerable for one reason or another. These populations are not fully granted rights to self-determination by the State, and instead others are authorized (parents, teachers, and so on) legitimately to override what might be incompetent or immature judgements.

A further, and crucial, point about the State's legitimate interference in the free choices of individuals relates to the harm that may be caused to others. All liberal accounts, and there are many, leave open a space for the intervention in people's private lives where innocent others will be harmed by the actions of an individual who pursues his or her own interests without proper regard for others. Intervention by the State, or others, over competent individuals is known as paternalism. In series of essays, liberal philosophers such as Ronald Dworkin (1972) and Joel Feinberg (1971, 1986) have argued that interventions over incompetent persons may be justified. Feinberg (1986) labels these acts of soft/weak paternalism. Like most liberals, however, he thought that interference in the lives of competent persons was typically unjustifiable. He calls this hard/strong paternalism.

What has all this to do with doping in sport? Well, a question remains as to *how* free individuals should be to prepare themselves for, and participate in, sporting competition. In other words, what kinds of limits are permitted both in the freedom to act and in the restrictions upon individual athletes? The interpretation of 'the spirit of sport' as a liberal view of human enhancement comes in several versions. Running the risk of simplification, we will distinguish between two forms here: the human enhancement view and the risk-reduction view.

An early criticism of the anti-doping campaign is found in the work of the American philosopher Miller Brown (1980, 1990). Sport is considered a cultural practice with the potential of realizing significant ethical values, among them empowerment of individuals as autonomous and responsible moral agents. Within competitions the rules of the game and norms of fair play are significant and ought to be kept. Outside of competitions, however, athletes ought to be free to choose the performance-enhancing means and methods they find appropriate and morally acceptable. Within the permissive paradigm, anti-doping regulations are expressions of anti-liberal views and of hard paternalism and counterproductive to the aim of moral development in sport. Among others Tamburrini (2000), Foddy and Savulescu (2007) and Savulescu *et al.* (2004) consider choice of performance-enhancing technologies as matters of individual, even professional, choice among athletes. From a similar position, Møller (2011) and Waddington (2011) present criticism against the WADA system of whereabouts information in which athletes have to report their daily whereabouts to be available for testing.

Philosophers such as Tamburrini and Savulescu take a further step and consider 'the spirit of sport' as an open sphere of human enhancement. They argue that human enhancement in terms of biomedically and genetically enhanced athletic performance should not merely be permissible as matters of free choice but are actually morally praiseworthy, and sports organizations should be tolerant of, and respect, this. Arguing from the twin premises of human freedom and the value of biotechnological possibilities to enhance human capabilities, they are open to the Promethean prospect of transcending problematic and limited aspects of human biology (Frannsen, 2013; McNamee 2007). Modern development within genetics is seen to carry particularly powerful potential. Proponents of liberal enhancement in medicine and biotechnology beyond sports envision not only physiological enhancement and increased longevity, but cognitive, social and moral enhancement as well (Agar, 2008; Harris, 2010; Savulescu 2007). Indeed, both Harris (2010) and Savulescu (2001) have proposed that individuals have a duty to enhance their children according to biotechnological possibilities with a view to bringing up – according to Savulescu (2001) – the best children possible. This has been viewed as a new form of eugenics (Sparrow, 2011), albeit within a liberal – not fascistic – world-view. Even one of its proponents (Agar, 2008) refers to this position as 'liberal eugenics' in an attempt to set it apart from its repressible political and military resonances of the recent past.

To liberal enhancement proponents, modern sport serves as a paradigmatic case. In sport, talented athletes set new records and transcend what were previously considered the limits of human potential. This, according to enhancement proponents, is the true nature or spirit of sport: a spirit of never-ending progress. As long as athletes can make informed choices, restrictions on their access to performance-enhancing substances and methods are in direct contradiction to this spirit. Doping rules and regulations appear as arbitrary interventions in the proper exercise of individual freedoms. Liberal enhancement proponents consider WADC distinctions between 'acceptable' and 'unacceptable' substances and methods as unjustifiable. Responsible and free choice and the use of performance-enhancing technologies are admirable and in line with the transcending spirit of sport and the potential benefits of human enhancement.

Liberal enhancement views are based on a very broad body of opinion and argument. Their adherents share many arguments and their positions are subtle and partly overlapping, while adhering to the general liberal position laid out at the beginning of this section. There is one further argument against anti-doping shared by many liberal enhancement proponents as well: the argument of harm reduction (Kayser *et al.*, 2007; Kayser and Smith 2008) that relates specifically to the second criterion of the WADC section on consideration for the Prohibited List. Whether one considers use of biomedical and biotechnological performance enhancement as acceptable, as with the liberal view, or as morally recommendable, as with the enhancement view, there is consensus on organized anti-doping work as a failure (Waddington, 2011). The large economic resources used to detect, deter and prevent use of banned substances and methods are considered as having meagre results. It is argued that athletes and support personnel engaged in doping practices are forced underground with significant costs in terms of increased health risks for athletes. Lifting the ban on performance-enhancing substances and methods – while at the same time installing responsible health surveillance for athletes – would be the superior approach.

The liberal enhancement interpretation of 'the spirit of sport' is contested. First, in particular, enhancement proponents are criticized by bio-conservatives (Schneider and Friedmann, 2006b; Kass, 2003; Murray, 2015; McNamee *et al.*, 2009; Loland, 2011) for holding a naïve view of the benefits and promises of new technologies. Even if developments of genetic technologies are promising, few gene-therapeutic techniques have been clinically cleared by regulatory authorities. Leading genetic scientists warn of complications, offering a modest picture of the state of the art than is propagated by commercial agencies (Schneider and Friedmann, 2006a; Bouchard and Hoffmann, 2011). In particular, genetic precursors of complex human skills and even cognitive and moral capabilities seem unrealistic. Complex capabilities, even more limited ones like sprinting, by their nature are not reducible to genetic profiles without remainder (Lucia *et al.*, 2007).

Further unanswered questions relate not so much to the state of cutting-edge biotechnology but to social and ethical questions regarding distributive justice. Who will get access to the benefits of potentially functional genetic and other biotechnological enhancements? Is there reason to believe that such enhancements will lead to even larger inequalities in society and in sport than is the case today? A final criticism concerns the very rationale for enhancement (Sandel, 2007). Why should we allow all kinds of biomedical and biotechnological performance enhancements in sport? If everyone enhances, where is the competitive advantage sought? And, if everyone is engaged in free enhancement projects, in what way would this make sport morally better? These questions remain largely unanswered in the permissive paradigm, whose goal is simply to maintain liberal freedoms and encourage a quest for enhancement.

The harm reduction view of the permissive paradigm has also been criticized. The portrayal of the anti-doping campaign appears as one-sided. Critics point to what they see as a common weakness among liberal enhancement views: they seem sociologically naïve (Loland, 2009a). Elite athletes start their careers early and are dependent upon external coaching and expertise. The ideal of free and informed choice of mature individuals when it comes to biomedical and biotechnological performance-enhancers is hard to realize. Moreover, the social logic of elite sport implies coaches and support systems who depend professionally upon sporting success (sometimes at whatever cost is thought necessary) (Green, 2009). After all, their jobs are on the line. As emphasized above, the incentives are strong for looking for substances and methods that provide even marginal competitive advantage. In such a context strong coercive pressures arise (Murray, 1983). Assumptions about free and informed choices among mature and autonomous athletes, and of responsible and harm reducing use of performance-enhancing substances and methods, seem unrealistic.

'The spirit of sport' as a restrictive view of development of human excellence

Permissive liberal views of human enhancement are not univocal. Neither are bio-conservative ones. Nevertheless, there is an identifiable group of interpretations of 'the spirit of sport' as the virtuous development of human excellence that lead to more restrictive views on doping and in most instances to support of the anti-doping campaign.

The dominant or official public sport policy response to biomedical performance-enhancing methods and substances is a restrictive one. WADA's references to 'the spirit of sport' are typical. Such positions strike important associations between sporting excellence and methods of preparation and competition and are ethically based, but are often left philosophically underdeveloped. From a systematic philosophical point of view, several scholars have proposed more elaborate interpretations.

The central premise of several of these approaches is that competitive sport is a sphere of ethically admirable human excellence. Sport is a cultural practice in which human capabilities of particular performances are measured, compared, and ranked (Loland, 2002). More generally, developing these capabilities is considered to lead towards moral development of the individual (McNamee *et al.*, 2003). The use of certain kinds of biomedical and biotechnological performance enhancement is considered counterproductive to moral development and generically labelled 'doping', to designate a pejorative stance (Fost, 2008; McNamee, 2009). One approach departs from an analysis of the logic of games and of sport as a cultural and social practice. An interconnected approach is a neo-Aristotelian understanding of human excellence. We will take a closer look at both and how they are combined.

In Bernard Suits' well-known analysis, playing a game is defined as a voluntary attempt to overcome unnecessary obstacles (Suits, 1978). Game rules define these obstacles; the rule against hand ball in soccer, against kicking the ball in handball, rules prescribing passing over the hurdles in a hurdle race and through the gates in a slalom race. According to Suits, such attempts are expressions of a lusory, or playful, attitude. In everyday or professional activities prohibiting the most efficient means to reach a goal seems irrational. The use of one's hands might be efficient if the point is to catch and control a ball. In normal life, where hurdles are in the way they are removed or avoided. In games, however, the voluntary attempt to overcome 'unnecessary obstacles' is the heart and soul of the enterprise: they make up their very meaning and value as they open for strong experiential qualities: fun, excitement, challenge, mastery and failure, a sense of community, and a sense of conflict. Games have the logic of autotelic activities. The logic of play is self-contained, not referring to external goals or attitudes.

From Plato via Huizinga to present-day philosophers of sport, such play is seen as having the potential of moral development as it is a clear expression of human freedom and possibility (Morgan, 2006). Most, though not all, draw more or less explicitly on Aristotelian ideals of human perfectibility. At its best, play can be an exponent of human excellence. In play, we explore who we are and might become (Reid, 2002). In sporting games, these explorations are done in embodied and concrete ways. The spirit of sport, Murray (2010, 2015) claims, is the virtuous development of natural talent towards human excellence.

The point here, and different from the liberal enhancement position, is that enhancement and performance development in sport has to take place in particular ways to enable development of virtue. What then are the criteria of the virtuous athlete? Here a catalogue of individual virtues has been proposed (Brown, 1980, 1990; McNamee, 1995; Reid, 2002; Jones, 2005). Others have approached the perspective of ethically admirable sports from a more system-oriented perspective (Loland, 2002). Perhaps the dominant appeal to ethically driven sport concerns itself with the ideas of fairness and justice.

A central argument in the doping debate is view of the use of certain biomedical and biotechnological performance-enhancing substances and methods as unfair. Indeed, the paradigmatic example is the use of prohibited means implying the covert breaking of anti-doping rules in order to gain an exclusive advantage. Use of these means is cheating. In a discussion of whether certain means and methods should be banned or not, however, the argument on cheating begs the question. One cannot justify a set of rules with reference to the wrongness of breaking them. As the liberals argue, one could remove the cheating argument in the blink of an eye by changing the rules that forbid those means and methods. A more fertile approach departs from ideas of institutional fairness and from what is referred to as the fair equality of opportunity principle (FEOP) (Loland, 2009b).

Where virtue ethicists draw on classic figures in ancient philosophy such as Aristotle, FEOP has a more modern provenance, drawing inspiration from the great eighteenth-century German philosopher Immanuel Kant and subsequent post-Kantian scholarship. One particular aspect is notable, in the ideal of never treating others as a mere means to our goals, but only and always also as persons worthy of respect in their own right. Thus in developed, democratic societies, FEOP lies at the core of distributing basic goods such as food, shelter, work, and to a certain extent income. Individuals with disabilities or with unfortunate setbacks in life are compensated. According to Loland (2002) the social structuring of sport reflects FEOP to a considerable extent. Classification schemes are designed to compensate for or eliminate inequalities that have impact on performance but that individuals cannot influence or control in any significant way: biological sex, body size in some sports, and age. Other inequalities, for instance inequalities in genetic predispositions for speed, endurance, power, or complex motor skills, are not compensated for, as these are inequalities that need to be developed through hard training and own efforts: that is, in an admirable and virtuous way.

Returning to the third WADC criterion of eligibility for the Prohibited List as violation against 'the spirit of sport', the question is whether biomedical and/or biotechnological enhanced performance ought to count as a proper constituent of athletic inequality, the very thing that sports contests should compare, measure, and rank. Proponents of the human excellence view argue in the negative. Use of substances and methods as those on the Prohibited List represents an externally administered enhancement of performance without requiring the relevant efforts and capabilities of the athlete. In varying degrees, responsibility for performance shifts from the athlete towards external expertise, and thus the admirable and virtuous basis of the performance is reduced or negated. Sport tends no longer to be an exponent of individual human excellence but increasingly becomes a struggle between overarching financial, scientific and technological systems in which the athlete is merely the top of the iceberg.

In addition, the restrictive position provides support to the health criterion. As noted above, it is true that elite sport in many cases is inherently linked to health risks, and to a certain extent to significant health risks, as in American football, boxing, ice hockey or rugby in which serious (including head) contact is foreseeable and frequent. Serious athletic training implies the risk of overtraining and fatigue injuries, intense competition can cause sudden injuries, some sports such as downhill skiing are inherently risky, with serious injury or even death as potential consequences of participation. Based on the human excellence criterion, however, the possibility is opened up to distinguish between relevant and non-relevant health risks (Loland, 2009a). The risk of training and competing hard without developing injuries is a challenge athletes have to face and handle themselves. Risk sports are among other things about athletes' capabilities of calculating and taking risks in responsible ways (Breivik, 2007). The risks involved in drug use, administered by external experts, into which most athletes do not have insights and upon which they have no control, do not contribute to athlete skill and mastery, nor to their empowerment as athletes or to human excellence. Hence, to proponents of the restrictive view, health risks linked to drug use can be considered non-relevant to sport. If 'the spirit of sport' refers to developing human excellence, a ban on certain performance-enhancing substances and methods makes sense and can be justified.

This conclusion should not be taken to imply that the approach from human excellence solves all problems involved in anti-doping. By and large the criticism of the anti-doping campaign referred to in the discussion of the liberal human enhancement view is itself a criticism of the restrictive human excellence approach. Although proponents of liberal human enhancement agree on the nature and social logic of sporting games and the necessity of fair play, they reject extending the restrictive logic outside of play. Moreover, their point of the difficulties of line drawing is relevant. The restrictive human excellence approach does not deliver ready-made solutions in difficult cases, such as the acceptability or non-acceptability of artificially constructed hypoxic conditions to enhance performance (Levine, 2006; Loland and Murray, 2007). To proponents of the restrictive view, however, this challenge is a sign of the debate over 'the spirit of sport' as authentic ethical terrain in which distinctions and lines are drawn by the use of example, reason and argument. Ethics is no exact science: it requires an ongoing discourse on the norms and values upon which human institutions, practices and actions are based. The restrictive human excellence approach is an attempt to articulate systematic and critical criteria to distinguish between acceptable and admirable athletic excellence from its simulacra.

Concluding comments

By looking critically at WADA's three potential criteria for deciding upon which substances and methods should be considered for the Prohibited List, we have argued that the basic issue and justification of anti-doping is a normative or value-laden one. Standpoints on the use of biomedical and biotechnological means to enhance performance in sport must necessarily be based on a vision of the nature and values of sport. Liberal or restrictive views are moral positions upon them.

WADA's third, normative criterion for substances and methods to be evaluated for the Prohibited List refers to 'the spirit of sport'. 'The spirit of sport', as we have shown, can be interpreted in several ways. With reference to the literature we have sketched two interpretations: what we have called the permissive liberal human enhancement interpretation and the restrictive human excellence interpretation. The two interpretations lead to contradictory conclusions for anti-doping: the liberal view is sometimes presented in such a way that it sees no justification for the anti-doping campaign, whereas in the restrictive human excellence view such a justification can be found. Which interpretation of 'the spirit of sport' seems to be the more reasonable one?

In our view, arguments from the liberal human enhancement camp do not provide sufficient answers to how biomedical and biotechnological enhancement adds sufficient value to the practice of sport. Moreover, compared to the human excellence approach, the liberal account seems to put less emphasis on the social power structures and the vulnerable position of individual athletes in elite sport.

Restrictive views (paradoxically) seem to lead to protection of athlete autonomy to a larger degree than liberal alternatives.

This does not mean that proponents of liberal and more restrictive views necessarily hold radically different views on the moral potential of sport. Most scholars on both sides of the doping debate share the vision of sport as a perfectionist sphere with positive ethical potential. There are, however, significant disagreements on the functions and consequences of the anti-doping campaign.

On a final note, we should bear in mind that the socio-cultural context of sport is in constant flux, and sociologically informed ethical and philosophical analyses must be revised accordingly. One possible future development is the overall general use of performance-enhancing technologies in both sport and society. If such use is based on informed consent and mature decisions, and if such use makes sport and more generally human life better and of higher quality, anti-doping justifications seem to lose force. As the situation is today, however, the burden of proof falls on proponents of a liberal view of legalizing. The weight of public authorities, sports bodies, the medical community, and the majority of athletes does not appear to side with them. Rather, a view of athletic enhancement understood within an overall view of human excellence in sport seems best realized within restrictive anti-doping regimes.

Note

1 https://wada-main-prod.s3.amazonaws.com/resources/files/wada-2015-world-anti-doping-code.pdf. Accessed 11 May 2015.

References

Agar, N. (2008). *Liberal Eugenics: In Defence of Human Enhancement*, London: John Wiley & Sons.

Bouchard, C. and Hoffman, E.P. (eds) (2011). *Genetic and Molecular Aspects of Sport Performance*, Oxford: Wiley-Blackwell.

Breivik, G. (2007). Can BASE Jumping be Morally Defended? In M.J. McNamee (ed.). *Philosophy, Risk and Adventure Sports*, Abingdon: Routledge.

Brown, W.M. (1980). Ethics, Drugs, and Sport. *Journal of the Philosophy of Sport*, 7 (1), 15–23.

Brown, W.M. (1990). Practices and Prudence. *Journal of the Philosophy of Sport*, 17 (1), 71–84.

Dworkin, G. (1972). Paternalism. *The Monist*, 64–84.

Feinberg, J. (1971). Legal Paternalism. *Canadian Journal of Philosophy*, 1 (1), 105–124.

Feinberg, J. (1986). *Harm to Self*, Oxford: Oxford University Press.

Foddy, B. and Savulescu, J. (2007). Ethics of Performance Enhancement in Sport: Drugs and Gene Doping. *Principles of Health Care Ethics*, second edition, Chichester: Blackwell Wiley, pp. 511–519.

Fost, N. (2008). 'Doping' is Pejorative and Misleading. *British Medical Journal*, 337, a910.

Franssen, T. (2013). Prometheus on Dope: A Natural Aim for Improvement or a Hubristic Drive to Mastery? In J. Tolleneer, S. Sterckx and P. Bonte (eds) *Athletic Enhancement, Human Nature and Ethics*, Dordrecht: Springer Netherlands, pp. 105–123.

Gleaves, J. and Llewellyn, M. (2014). Sport, Drugs, and Amateurism: Tracing the Real Cultural Origins of Anti-Doping Rules in International Sport. *The International Journal for the History of Sport*, 31 (8), 839–853.
Green, G.A. (2009). The Role of Physicians, Scientists, Trainers, Coaches, and other Nonathletes in Athletes' Drug Use. In T.H. Murray, K.J. Maschke and A.A. Wasunna (eds) *Performance-enhancing Technologies in Sport. Ethical, Conceptual and Scientific Issues*, Baltimore: Johns Hopkins University Press, pp. 81–95.
Harris, J. (2010) *Enhancing Evolution. The Ethical Case for Making Better People*, Princeton, NJ: Princeton University Press.
Jones, C. (2005). Character, Virtue and Physical Education. *European Physical Education Review*, 11(2), 139–151.
Jones, C. and McNamee, M. (2000). Moral Reasoning, Moral Action, and the Moral Atmosphere of Sport. *Sport, Education and Society*, 5 (2), 131–146.
Kass, L.R. (2003). *Beyond Therapy: Biotechnology and the Pursuit of Happiness*, New York: Dana Press.
Kayser, B. and Smith, A.C.T. (2008). Globalisation of Anti-doping: The Reverse Side of the Medal. *British Medical Journal*, 337, 584.
Kayser, B., Mauron, A. and Miah, A. (2007). Current Anti-doping Policy: A Critical Appraisal. *BMC Medical Ethics*, 8 (1), 2.
Levine, B. (2006). Should Artificial High Altitude Environments Be Considered Doping? *Scandinavian Journal of Medicine and Science in Sports*, 16, 297–301.
Loland, S. (2002). *Fair Play. A Moral Norm System*, London: Routledge.
Loland, S. (2009a). The Ethics of Performance-enhancing Technology in Sport. *Journal of the Philosophy of Sport*, XXXVI (2), s. 152–161.
Loland, S. (2009b). Fairness in Sport: An Ideal and Its Consequences. In T.H. Murray, K.J. Maschke and A.A. Wasunna (eds) *Performance-enhancing Technologies in Sport. Ethical, Conceptual and Scientific Issues*, Baltimore: Johns Hopkins University Press, pp. 160–174.
Loland, S. (2011). Genetics and Ethics in Elite Sport. In C. Bouchard and E.P. Hoffman (eds) *Genetic and Molecular Aspects of Sport Performance*, Oxford: Wiley-Blackwell, pp. 353–360.
Loland, S. and Murray, T.H. (2007). The Ethics of the Use of Technologically Constructed High-altitude Environments to Enhance Performance in Sport. *Scandinavian Journal of Medicine and Science in Sport*, 17 (3), 193–195.
Lucia, A., Oliván, J., Gómez-Gallego, F., Santiago, C., Montil, M. and Foster, C. (2007). Citius and Longius (faster and longer) with No α-actinin-3 in Skeletal Muscles? *British Journal of Sports Medicine*, 41(9), 616–617.
McNamee, M.J. (1995). Sporting Practices, Institutions, and Virtues: A Critique and a Restatement. *Journal of the Philosophy of Sport*, 22(1), 61–82.
McNamee, M.J. (2007). Whose Prometheus? Transhumanism, Biotechnology and the Moral Topography of Sports Medicine. *Sports, Ethics and Philosophy*, 1 (2), 181–194.
McNamee, M.J. (2008). *Sports, Virtues and Vices: Morality Plays*, London: Routledge.
McNamee, M.J. (2012). The Spirit of Sport and the Medicalisation of Anti-doping: Empirical and Normative Ethics. *Asian Bioethics Review*, 4 (4), 374–392.
McNamee, M.J., Jones, C. and Duda, J.L. (2003). Psychology, Ethics and Sports. *International Journal of Sport and Health Science*, 1 (1), 61–75.
McNamee, M.J., Müller, A., van Hilvoorde, I. and Holm, S. (2009). Genetic Testing and Sports Medicine Ethics. *Sports Medicine*, 39 (5), 339–344.
Mill, J.S. (1859). *On Liberty*, Oxford: Oxford University Press.

Møller, V. (2011). *The Scapegoat. About the Expulsion of Michael Rasmussen from Tour de France in 2007 and Beyond*, Aarhus: Akaprint.
Morgan, W.J. (2006). *Why Sports Morally Matter*, New York: Routledge.
Murray, T.H. (1983). The Coercive Power of Drugs in Sport. *The Hastings Center Report*, XIII, s. 24–30.
Murray, T.H. (2007). Enhancement. In B. Steinbock (ed.) *The Oxford Handbook of Bioethics*, Oxford: Oxford University Press, pp. 491–515.
Murray, T.H. (2010). Preserving Sporting Values and Ethics: The Relationship between Anti-doping and Sport Values and Ethics; available at: http://unesdoc.unesco.org/images/0018/001884/188404e.pdf. Accessed 25 May 2015.
Murray, T.H. (2015). Doping and Anti-doping: An Enquiry into the Meaning of Sport. In M.J. McNamee and W. Morgan (eds) *Routledge Handbook of the Philosophy of Sport*, Abingdon: Routledge, pp. 315–332.
Reid, H. L. (2002). *The Philosophical Athlete*, Durham, NC: Carolina Academic Press.
Sandel, M. (2007). *The Case Against Perfection. Ethics in the Age of Genetic Engineering*, Cambridge, MA: Belknap Press.
Savulescu, J. (2001). Procreative Beneficence: Why We Should Select the Best Children. *Bioethics*, 15 (5–6), 413–426.
Savulescu, J. (2007). Genetic Interventions and the Ethics of Enhancement of Human Beings. In B. Steinbock (ed.) *The Oxford Handbook of Bioethics*, Oxford: Oxford University Press, pp. 516–535.
Savulescu, J., Foddy, B. and Clayton, M. (2004). Why We Should Allow Performance-enhancing Drugs in Sport. *British Journal of Sport Medicine*, 38, 666–670.
Schneider, A.J. and Friedmann, T. (2006a). Gene Doping in Sports: The Science and Ethics of Genetically Modified Athletes. *Adv. Genet.* 51, 1–110.
Schneider, A.J. and Friedmann, T. (2006b). Gene Transfer in Sports: An Opening Scenario for Genetic Enhancement of Normal 'Human Traits'. *Advances in Genetics*, 51, 37–49.
Sparrow, R. (2011). A Not-So-New Eugenics. *Hastings Center Report*, 41 (1), 32–42.
Suits, B. (1978). *Grasshopper: Games, Life and Utopia*. Toronto: University of Toronto Press.
Tamburrini, C.M. (2000). What's Wrong with Doping? In T. Tännsjö and C.M. Tamburrini (eds) *Values in Sport: Elitism, Nationalism, Gender Equality and the Scientific Manufacture of Winners*, Abingdon: Routledge, pp. 200–216.
Waddington, I. (2011). 'A Prison of Measured Time?' A Sociologist Looks at the WADA Whereabouts System. In M.J. McNamee and V. Moller (eds) *Doping and Anti-Doping Policy in Sport: Ethical, Legal and Social Perspectives*, Abingdon: Routledge, pp. 183–199.

9 The ethics of doping from a public health perspective

Thomas H. Murray

The case for sport free from the distortions of performance enhancing drugs is not quite so self-evident as many lovers of clean sport might hope. Along with the scientists who devise doping methods, the enablers who provide doping technologies and urge or pressure athletes to use them, and the athletes who succumb, there are those who oppose anti-doping on a number of grounds.

Some of the critics seize on what they claim are the flaws of anti-doping programs; others argue that the use of performance enhancing drugs by athletes is either ethically permissible or even admirable. A brief survey of the most important arguments offered by anti-doping skeptics will provide the background against which the case against doping in sport must be made.

The ethical defense of anti-doping and its critics

The ethical foundation of anti-doping rests on three principles: Promote fairness; Protect health; and Preserve meaning. Fairness requires assuring that no athlete has an unfair advantage over his or her competitors. Anti-doping programs attempt to ensure fairness. Fairness of a kind, however, might also be achieved by allowing all athletes to use performance enhancing technologies, or so some critics claim. The deeper critique of doping in sport must therefore be found in the other two principles: Protect health and Preserve meaning.

Protecting health, in particular, is a problem in public health ethics, as I discovered more than three decades ago when I first began listening to athletes and others with intimate knowledge of elite sport. When I asked why an athlete would use a drug such as a synthetic anabolic steroid or an amphetamine, the answer was clear: Athletes fear that their competitors are using those very drugs and thereby gaining a competitive advantage. If athletes don't want to lose to someone who may be less talented and less dedicated, they may feel they must resort to using the same performance enhancing drugs as their competitors.[1]

Why is this a matter for public health ethics and not simply the choices of individuals? Norman Fost, one of the early critics of anti-doping, said this in 1986: "Whether or not a competent person seeks pleasure or financial gain involving risk is a personal decision. So long as the activity is not imposing burdens involuntarily on others, we reject paternalistic interference with risky behavior."[2] [p. 7] His article was in response to one I had published three years earlier in which I described the great pressures athletes experienced to use performance enhancing drugs in order to avoid giving up a critical competitive edge. At that time I wrote:

> When a young person has devoted years to reach the highest levels in an event, only to find that to compete successfully he or she must take potentially grave risks to health, we have as serious a threat to human flourishing as many restrictions on liberty.
>
> [p. 29]

Fost was not persuaded. He distinguished between an *offer* and a *threat*. A threat is coercive and therefore an affront to individual liberty. But, to him, the situation faced by athletes, including young athletes, was merely an offer. I believed then, and I believe now, that this view fails to understand the circumstances of young aspiring athletes. It also trivializes the intense pressures they can experience to use doping technologies. USADA's investigation of cycling tore the curtain off the charade that professional road cycling had choreographed. Its "Reasoned Decision" recounted the experiences of many athletes who had been seduced by a culture that not merely condoned doping but systematically normalized doping, provided the materials and expertise, and effectively demanded that young cyclists get with the program or leave.[3] Some did leave. But many succumbed. To see this elaborate process of enculturation to doping as merely an "offer" is simplistic and naïve.

Impact of a culture of doping on athletes

Jonathan Vaughters raced in the Tour de France as Lance Armstrong's teammate. He is now Manager of the Cannondale-Garmin team. In the *New York Times* he described the choice a talented, ambitious young cyclist faced in an era when doping was endemic: "Almost every athlete I've met who has doped will say they did it only because they wanted a level playing field. That says something: everyone wants a fair chance, not more." The choice was not a simple one, like deciding whether to go to a movie Saturday evening. Vaughters again: "Young cyclists' identities were intimately tied up with success in their sport. In many instances they had foregone other life opportunities to concentrate on this one avenue."[4]

What happens to elite athletes who refuse to dope? Bradley McGee, an Australia Olympic track cyclist and Tour de France competitor, has this to say about his experience:

> I was competing not just against Armstrong, but against the Armstrong years. I feel my professional years – my Tour de France years – have been stolen.... The more I think about it, the more it makes me mad as hell. But I have to move on from the fact that I have, more than likely, missed out on results and revenue, plus more, because of others' doping.[5]

Scott Mercier was a member of the US Postal team in May 1997 when he was summoned to the hotel room of the team's physician. This is his account of what happened:

> [The physician] handed me a bag containing a bottle of green pills and several vials of clear liquid … I was given a 17-day training schedule too. Each day had either a dot or a star. A dot represented a pill and a star was an injection. He said: "They're steroids, you go strong like bull." Then he said: "Put it in your pocket, if you get stopped at customs say it's B vitamins." That was when I decided I didn't want to be a pro cyclist any more. I got home and decided: "No, thank you." I love cycling, it's a beautiful sport, but it would have been very difficult for me to look anyone in the eye and say I was clean when I wasn't.[6]

What the critics say

Critics of anti-doping are quick to point out that prohibiting athletes from using performance enhancing technologies can be interpreted as a form of paternalism – doing something to or for a person to advance their welfare but without regard for that person's values and preferences. If that were the whole of the story this justification for anti-doping would collapse except for child and adolescent athletes for whom paternalism can be defended. However, multiple features in the structure of competitive sport make it clear that the decision to use a performance enhancing technology is profoundly shaped by many external factors and affects other persons acutely, not merely the individual making that decision. Recent work in public health ethics provides conceptual tools for analyzing what it means to protect health in the case of performance enhancing drugs in sport. Before turning to those analytical resources it will be helpful to review the major lines of attack employed by critics of anti-doping.

Pro-doping vs. anti-anti-doping

Criticisms of anti-doping can be grouped into two broad categories: pro-doping and the unfortunately awkward label of anti-anti-doping.[7] Many anti-doping critics deploy both types of arguments, but it's useful to keep in mind the distinction. Pro-doping arguments see nothing wrong with using performance enhancing technologies such as anabolic steroids or EPO in sport. Some advocates of the pro-doping position see doping as morally neutral or inconsequential; others see it as a morally positive thing. For example, Savulescu and colleagues say this:

> Far from being against the spirit of sport, biological manipulation embodies the human spirit – the capacity to improve ourselves on the basis of reason and judgment. When we exercise our reason, we do what only humans do.… Sport would be less of a genetic lottery. The winner will be the person

> with a combination of the genetic potential, training, psychology, and judgment.[8]

In a similar vein, Miah describes a (fictitious) swimmer with surgically enhanced webbing in fingers and toes and calls for us to

> celebrate the rise of a new age of genuinely superhuman athletes, where the rules of sports are governed not by ever-present but ultimately unreliable doping police, but by a genuine concern for optimizing excellence. As technology gets better, athletes should, too.[9]

The phrase "optimizing excellence" illuminates the sensibilities underlying pro-doping. "Optimizing" suggests computer routines, mathematical functions or business processes. It connotes technological paths to achieving maximal performance. The term "excellence," on the other hand, simply begs the question. What form(s) of excellence are we hoping to advance and celebrate here? The surgeon's skill at constructing webs between fingers and toes? The pharmacist's ability to create drug regimens that increase strength and endurance? Or the athlete's dedication to perfecting her talents? All these factors affect how quickly a swimmer completes a race, as does the type of suit she wears. But the sport of swimming banned many suits even though they led to faster times.[10] What could justify banning technologies that improve performance? Clearly, swimming has a different understanding of excellence than that assumed by pro-doping enthusiasts.

Though scholars advancing pro-doping arguments may disagree with each other at times about precisely which biomedical enhancements ought to be permitted, the core of pro-doping appears to be a conviction that such technological enhancements are desirable because they advance some good such as improved performance, a more level playing field, or individual liberty. If they are indeed effective, biomedical enhancements certainly accomplish the first item in the list – improved performance. But Savulescu's claim that enhancing athletic performance by any and all biological manipulations is the real spirit of sport is far from self-evident. Consider the revised 2015 WADA Code's description of the "spirit of sport":

> it is the essence of Olympism, the pursuit of human excellence through the dedicated perfection of each person's natural talents. It is how we play true. The spirit of sport is the celebration of the human spirit, body and mind, and is reflected in values we find in and through sport.[11]

The emphasis on perfecting one's *natural* talents highlights two key differences between the meaning of sport implicit in the WADA Code versus the assumptions of pro-doping advocates. The first has to do with the means of "perfecting" one's talents. Many technological shortcuts, from drugs such as anabolic steroids and stimulants to EPO and human growth hormone, are banned by WADA on the grounds that they are just that – shortcuts – and therefore *illegitimate* paths around the tasks essential to becoming a successful athlete: training; practice; studying one's sport; all the elements that transform raw talent into outstanding performance. Loland and Hoppeler put the distinction this way:

> Most substances and methods on the doping list are qualitatively different because they bypass the body's natural and evolutionary based complex stress and compensation reactions. The use of prohibited substances and methods overruns natural talent, reduces athletes' possibilities of developing sporting excellence as human excellence in virtuous ways, and contradicts the spirit of sport.[12]
>
> [p. 352]

The second difference has to do with which particular human talents are regarded as relevant for sport. Sport traditionally recognizes – indeed, celebrates – differences in natural talents, particularly physical talents such as strength, speed, leaping ability, reaction time and the like. This leaves ample room for other talents such as dedication, intelligence, self-discipline and other human capacities. The pro-doping arguments, on the other hand, appear to see differences in human talents, especially physical capacities, as a problem to be solved by technology. Savulescu and colleagues imagine that biomedical enhancement will attenuate what they call the "genetic lottery." They prefer that athletic success be due to training, psychology and judgment rather than natural talents. Of course training, psychology and judgment are likewise embraced by supporters of doping-free sport. The contention is over how to think about differences in natural talents.

Tamburrini welcomes genetic enhancement of athletes claiming that "genetic modifications probably will level out differences in performance capacity established by birth." He argues that such leveling will make competitions fairer. He asserts there will be "more room for morality in this enhanced new (sport) world." Outcomes in this new world of sport will depend more on "moral and intellectual excellence (effort, willingness to pursuit [sic] a goal and the mental strength and capacity to achieve it etc.)"[13] Differences in physical talents in this view are wellsprings of unfairness, not forms of human excellence to be perfected and celebrated. Advocates of doping-free sport would no doubt embrace moral and intellectual excellences. But they are unlikely to see differences in athletic talents as inherently unfair.

Anti-anti-doping

Anti-anti-doping arguments, rather than focusing on the moral desirability or acceptability of doping, instead focus on alleged flaws with current anti-doping policies and practices. Critics raise a variety of issues, five of which warrant discussion here: conceptual ambiguities; possible injustices; cost and effectiveness; privacy; and redirecting the goal of anti-doping toward harm reduction.

Conceptual ambiguities

Why does sport accept certain technologies but reject others? Can a coherent distinction be drawn between them? Anti-doping skeptics have long expressed doubt that such a conceptually coherent line can be drawn.[14] In the past, critics have asked why EPO is prohibited but training at high altitude is not, given that both are ways to raise hematocrit levels and increase endurance. More recently, they have added to the mix hypoxic chambers, which allow athletes to train near sea level but spend the remainder of their time in an oxygen-depleted environment simulating high elevations.[15] Defenders of doping-free sport note that sport must continually draw lines along continua in order to create meaningful competitions, whether it be the dimensions of the playing field or goal or the types of equipment athletes use.[16] They acknowledge that defensible lines can be difficult to draw at times.[17] But they strive also to offer principled defenses of such distinctions.[12] In the end, critics confuse the ever-present conceptual challenges faced by sport in deciding what to permit and what to prohibit with an indefensible conceptual muddle. Sport must be very clear about its reasons for drawing lines in particular places, and must have a defensible process for making such decisions. In the absence of sound principles and process, sport is indeed liable to fall into the conceptual muddle its critics decry.

Possible injustices

Justice requires treating like cases alike and different cases differently. There can be no doubt that current anti-doping measures fall short, though not in the direction that evokes the loudest complaints – from athletes who swear they were falsely accused of doping. The system is designed to avoid punishing innocent athletes. If an error is made in collecting urine or blood, the chain of custody is not pristine, or the laboratory analysis is not iron-clad, a doping athlete is likely to escape sanction. Athletes have the right to appeal to the Council of Arbitration for Sport if they claim any irregularities or unfairness. On the other side, we know that doping athletes have escaped detection, sometimes for many years.[3] This is both defect and design feature.[18] The very high bar set for sanctioning an athlete for doping means that some will surely evade justice – at least for a time. The athletes who suffer most from injustice are those who compete clean and, as a consequence, lose out to others who dope. The *raison d'être* for anti-doping is to provide reasonable assurance that the playing field is indeed level. Treating like cases alike would include sanctions on all who dope; sport is far away from that goal. But the panoply of anti-doping activities, which include education, efforts to change the environment in which athletes live and learn and to reform the culture of sport, as well as testing, are meant to bring sport closer to the goal.

Cost and effectiveness

Are the resources devoted to anti-doping worth the expense or are they wasted? Are they deployed in the most effective ways or could they be redirected to achieve the same goals more efficiently? Some critics point to the persistence of doping among athletes as evidence that resources are wasted on anti-doping programs.[19] But critics do not agree with anti-doping defenders either on the goals of such programs or on how to gauge success. If the goals of anti-doping programs are those described above – promoting fairness, protecting health and preserving meaning – the critics are prone to dismiss the first (by noting that if all athletes had access to the same performance enhancing drugs the field would be, in a way, level), reinterpret the second (by allowing "safe" drugs and putting doctors in charge of managing athletes' doping) and ignore the third. There are good reasons to doubt whether athletes' health would in fact be protected better if we followed the critics' advice. The disagreement over the meaning of sport, however, may be even more fundamental. Both of these will be addressed later.

How should we gauge success? The standard lies somewhere along a continuum with absolutely no use of banned performance enhancing technologies anchoring one end, and being able to compete with reasonable confidence that your competitors are not gaining a meaningful advantage over you by using such technologies on the other end. Appreciating the fallibility of human beings, and understanding the pressures placed on athletes to succeed, it seems unreasonable to require anti-doping programs to achieve perfection and to judge anything short of that as abysmal failure. What level of imperfection is tolerable for such a program to be defensible is of course open to debate. When cyclists say that they believe they can now compete without doping and have a chance to succeed based on their talent and dedication, we have evidence that anti-doping efforts are making an impact.

In all cases, anti-doping programs must be responsible stewards of the resources entrusted to them. They should exercise great care to use those resources responsibly, effectively and efficiently.

Privacy

People who are not elite athletes might well find it odd to have someone observing them as they urinate. And unless they are the subjects of a formal monitoring program, they are unlikely to be providing details of their present and future whereabouts to strangers. Yet athletes who wish to compete in the Olympics or any other sport that follows WADA's standards for anti-doping are expected to submit to both kinds of intrusions on their privacy. What could justify such measures? In the first place there must be some organic connection to justifiable, shared goals that require these intrusions on privacy. It would also be good if the individuals whose privacy was at issue consented to or, better, approved of these practices.

So-called "observed voiding" was instituted once it was discovered that some athletes who were asked to provide samples of their urine for testing proved to be very creative in substituting other fluids through means up to and including fake penises. Watching the athlete as he or she fills the sample jar makes substitution far more difficult.

Whereabouts reporting is a more recent development in response to the reality that some of the most effective performance enhancing drugs such as EPO and anabolic steroids exert their effect during training; all traces may be gone by the time the athlete shows up to compete. To discourage the use of drugs during training we need some way of determining who might be using them at that time. Out-of-competition testing is one strategy, but its success depends upon knowing where the athlete is so that the doping control officer can find the athlete. From those circumstances the whereabouts program was born. Critics have decried it as a violation of human rights.[20]

Athletes have at times bemoaned its impact on their lives and the enjoyment of their sport.[21] However, as that same survey of Danish athletes showed, most of them accepted it; some regarded it as a compliment of sorts – an acknowledgement of their status as elite athletes. Other studies have found considerable support among athletes including calls to strengthen it by making out-of-competition testing even less predictable and more comprehensive.[22] In any event, athletes who desire to compete in the Olympics, say, know that whereabouts programs and observed voiding are a condition for their eligibility. Critics may argue that such conditions are unjustified intrusions on athletes' privacy, that athletes should have the choice to compete without subjecting themselves to such intrusions, and that their consent cannot bear the moral weight placed on it. Public health ethics deals regularly with balancing individuals' privacy against other important goods. We will look more closely at whereabouts testing after gleaning whatever insights we can from the literature on public health ethics.

Redirecting anti-doping toward harm reduction

Perhaps the most creative attack on anti-doping has been the suggestion that drugs in sport be treated as a public health problem similar to heroin or other drugs of abuse. Harm reduction strategies such as needle exchanges have had success in reducing disease transmission among injecting-drug users. Why not, some critics have proposed, allow "low harm" drugs in sport and shift the focus of testing from deterring all use to merely protecting against harmful use?[23] As desirable is the goal of reducing harm, this proposal encounters several difficulties.

First, discerning which drugs are "low harm" in the context of sport's quest for performance enhancement turns out to be difficult. In a key article advancing the proposal, anabolic steroids are mentioned as an example of a class of drugs that could be managed in a harm reduction program. Some scholars claim that the risks of anabolic steroids are exaggerated.[24] Others who review the evidence conclude that the risks are substantial.[25] EPO, another candidate for "low harm," has been linked to increased risks of death, stroke, heart attack and blood clots – sufficient for the US Food and Drug Administration to require a "black box" warning on its packaging.[26]

Second, while the goal of protecting athletes from harm is important, it is not the only goal of anti-doping. Preserving meaning is also one of the central justifications. If these two goals were in direct opposition should a harm reduction program be instituted in sport, we might face a difficult decision. But the analogy between harm reduction strategies for drugs of abuse and for performance enhancing drugs in sport is fatally flawed. There is good reason to think that the overall risk of harm would not be reduced and might even increase. The analogies to public health ethics are particularly helpful here.

If certain anabolic steroids, EPO or other performance enhancing drugs are declared "safe" and made available to athletes they will immediately constitute the floor – the essential list of drugs all athletes must take to remain competitive in whatever sport those drugs confer competitive advantage. Everything we know about the incentives structuring athletes' behavior tells us that some will immediately try to leap above that floor by taking larger doses of the permitted drugs and adding additional, banned drugs to their regimen. Other athletes will be compelled to compete at a disadvantage or join in the above-the-floor drug-taking, replicating the same dynamic that led to anti-doping programs in the first place.

In addition, there is every reason to think that use of at least the permitted drugs will increase among non-elite athletes. Young people in particular strive to emulate the athletes they admire by using the same bikes, shoes, jerseys, etc. Now they will also want to use the same drugs – except that they may have to resort to less secure and reliable channels to obtain the drugs – think online pharmacies peddling drugs across borders with little or no assurance that the drugs are pure or safe. Further, if such non-elite, aspiring athletes have medical management at all, it is likely to be less expert and more sporadic. This is contagion of a kind, analogous to that encountered in public health contexts. It's hard to see how spreading the use of powerful drugs such as anabolic steroids and EPO among a much larger, more naïve and fitfully monitored population could be benign.

The problem lies in the fatally flawed analogy with harm reduction strategies for drugs of abuse. To put it simply, heroin addicts do not compete with one another to see who can get "higher." But that is precisely what athletes do. If we raise the floor, no athlete will want to allow her competitor to occupy it without clambering up there herself. And the proposal does nothing to disrupt the dynamic that drives athletes to seek advantages while putting other athletes in the awful position of having to choose whether to cede competitive advantage, drop out of the competition or give in and use the same drugs.

Advocates for the harm reduction approach to drugs in sport suggest "testing for health" in place of testing for the presence of banned drugs, and placing the management of each athlete's drug use with his or her physician. Elite athletes are typically under intense medical scrutiny already, but precisely how will their physicians "test for health" while athletes are taking potent performance enhancing drugs? Will the tools available to physicians enable them to identify deleterious health consequences early enough to intervene? Some serious consequences, such as the strokes, heart attacks and blood clots caused by EPO, may erupt too suddenly to detect and prevent. If any of the drug regimens athletes are on are causing long-term health risks, their physicians may simply be unable to see the early signs in time. Many cancers, for example, have long latency periods. The perturbations of anatomy (for example, the masculinization of secondary sex characteristics among female users of anabolic steroids) and physiology (for example, liver function in anabolic steroids) may persist for years, decades or a lifetime.[27] "Testing for health" may allow physicians to see what they can see today, but there is no guarantee that all significant risks, immediate or long term, could be detected or prevented.

Then there is the problem that physicians entrusted with athletes' health do not always act to protect the athletes under their care. The notorious state-organized doping program in East Germany enlisted many physicians and scientists.[28] The history of elite sport is rife with examples of physicians who aided and abetted athletes' doping.[29] In some notorious cases, physicians designed doping programs for athletes. There are undoubtedly many ethical physicians who would take the responsibility of managing athletes' health seriously. But the role physicians play in sport is not always in a traditional physician–patient relationship; they may have a conflicting loyalty to a team, owner, league or government.[30]

In the end, the proposal to "test for health" and entrust doping management to physicians fails to inspire confidence for all the reasons just described. But neither does it solve the problems it presumably set out to deal with. The fundamental dynamic driving performance enhancing drug use in sport remains completely intact. Unless the proposed measures could dismantle or defeat that powerful dynamic, there would continue to be a need for some system to deter performance enhancing drug use above the permitted floor. What that system might look like, how it might differ from the current system of education, testing, adjudication and sanction, and whether it would have a net advantage, is unclear. Advocates for such an alternative have yet to make a persuasive case.

Doping control as a problem in public health ethics

Public health measures typically involve governments exercising control over certain aspects of people's lives or gathering information about them. As a consequence, discussions about ethics and public health typically assume that the entity asserting authority is a government. Although government agencies may become involved in one or another aspect of doping control, the overarching entities in sport are non-governmental agencies such as the IOC, the various international federations such as IAAF, FINA or UCI, and WADA, along with national anti-doping agencies. Understanding the implications of public health ethics for doping control, therefore, will require some translation. But the issues are sufficiently similar that it will be helpful to assess anti-doping programs against the highest standards of public health ethics.

Faden and Shebaya describe a key task of public health ethics as

> determining self-imposed limitations and restrictions on what can reasonably come under the auspices of public health authorities, for reasons having

> to do with concerns about individual liberty, about privacy and paternalism, about democratic process, and about the place of health in relation to other aspects of human well-being.[31]

Kass lists similar concerns:

> Although a variety of burdens or harms might exist in public health programs, the majority will fall into 3 broad categories: risks to privacy and confidentiality, especially in data collection activities; risks to liberty and self-determination, given the power accorded public health to enact almost any measure necessary to contain disease; and risks to justice, if public health practitioners propose targeting public health interventions only to certain groups.[32]

The most obvious shared challenges for anti-doping programs have to do with liberty, privacy and confidentiality, and democratic process, understood in this context as reasonable representation of the views of those most affected, namely the athletes. Justice would be an issue if the burdens of anti-doping were shown to fall disproportionately on certain groups, particularly disadvantaged groups, with no good reason. Faden and Shebaya's concern about the place of health in relation to other aspects of human well-being appears to be motivated by the worry that protecting health will be over-valued at the expense of other forms of human flourishing. This does not appear to be the case with elite sport.

Consider liberty. An athlete's freedom to use a performance enhancing drug (for the moment, assume that the drug is legal and would otherwise be legitimately obtainable by the athlete) is clearly infringed by anti-doping rules prohibiting such use. What could justify this infringement on liberty? If we said we were doing it for that athlete's own good, despite her preferences otherwise, it would be a clear instance of paternalism. Now, under certain circumstances, say very young athletes, paternalism can be justified. But it's a hard case to make. Fortunately, we don't need to make it here because the primary reason for infringing on any particular athlete's liberty is to protect the well-being of his or her fellow athletes. This follows from the structure of sport and the powerful dynamic that motivates each athlete not to give up a competitive advantage. To the extent that an athlete is confident that his or her competitors are not getting an advantage from banned performance enhancing drugs, the pressure to use them diminishes.

Practices such as observed voiding, whereabouts requirements and so-called "knock-and-pee" testing surely infringe on privacy and confidentiality. In light of deceptive tactics used to avoid giving one's own sample, and the prevalence and significance of drugs used during training, these practices have at least a prima facie rationale. If we ceased observed voiding, cheaters would have an easy time providing fake urine samples. If we stopped testing athletes away from competitions, dishonest athletes could use many of the most effective performance enhancing drugs with no worry about being detected. This is not, however, a complete defense. What other tests should an intrusive measure such as a whereabouts program meet?

Justifying public health interventions

Childress and Bernheim describe five justificatory conditions for public health interventions.[33] The first condition is *effectiveness*. They note that: "interventions that infringe important social values must have a reasonable prospect of success in order to be justified." A whereabouts program that had no deterrent effect would be unjustifiable. Whether, in fact, current whereabouts programs are effective is an empirical question. That would appear to confer an obligation on anti-doping programs to assess their effectiveness, and to pursue strategies such as continuous quality improvement in order to maximize effectiveness.

The second condition is *necessity*. They offer this observation: "Liberty and other presumptive values require a search for alternatives before they can be justifiably overridden." Are there other, less intrusive ways to deter performance enhancing drug use outside of competition? If, for example, we could determine who used EPO, steroids or growth hormone through residues in hair, this would be a far gentler impingement on privacy. In the absence of less intrusive alternatives, whereabouts programs may be justifiable. Anti-doping programs should work to develop less intrusive methods wherever possible.

Their third condition insists that the intervention constitute the *least infringement of presumptive value* consistent with the achievement of the legitimate public health goal. They observe:

> even if it is justifiable to breach privacy or confidentiality in particular circumstances, this third condition places limits on the scope of the infringement, in terms of both the information that is disclosed and the parties to whom it is disclosed.

This condition implies that whereabouts programs should gather no more information that is absolutely necessary for their effective implementation, and that the confidentiality of whatever information is collected must be scrupulously protected.

Proportionality is their fourth condition. In the context of quarantine they write:

> After determining that a proposed coercive intervention such as quarantine would satisfy the first three conditions, we still have to ask whether the probable benefits (in risk reduction), minus any probable negative effects, are sufficient to rebut the presumption in favor of freedom from governmental coercion.

Are the benefits of whereabouts programs, minus their negative effects, sufficient to rebut the presumption in favor of privacy? Athletes appear to think so as documented previously. As circumstances evolve, however, the proportionality test should be reapplied.

The final condition is *impartiality*: "Basic standards of fairness apply across public health interventions. More specifically, they require that coercive public health measures ... be imposed impartially." The concern here is with stigmatization and discrimination, which have been known to mar public health interventions but don't appear to be a problem with whereabouts programs in anti-doping. Nevertheless, we should remain vigilant against the possibility of violating impartiality.

On the whole, and in light of what evidence we have, whereabouts programs appear to satisfy the five conditions Childress and Bernheim propose to evaluate the ethics of public health interventions. These helpful criteria, though, are reminders to those who design, manage and execute such programs of their continuing ethical obligations to insure that the program is effective, necessary, the least infringement possible, proportionate and impartial.

Faden and Shebaya had one additional relevant standard: a democratic process. Athletes in certain professional leagues such as the NBA, NFL and MLB have unions empowered to negotiate with team owners and league officials. Amateur athletes typically lack such sources of collective power. All the more important then to assure that athletes' representatives have standing in the rule-making and enforcing bodies of sport, that athletes' voices are sought and respected, and that anti-doping be responsive to the insights and concerns athletes are especially well placed to offer, and that athletes above all must live with.

Meanings and values in sport

Beyond providing a fair and level playing field, and protecting athletes' health, anti-doping programs should strive to preserve meaning and to support those values we find in and through sport. If the critics are correct, the meaning of sport is to optimize performance, or as Savulescu and colleagues assert: "in many ways the athletic ideal of modern athletes is inspired by the myth of the marathon. Their ideal is superhuman performance, at any cost."[34] But there is good reason to doubt that the critics' version is correct. Individual sports regularly reject equipment that makes it easier to do whatever that sport deems important. Swimming rejects buoyant, super-slippery swimsuits, golf rejects balls that fly straighter and clubs that diminish the difficulty of hitting out of the rough. And virtually all sports reject the use of performance enhancing drugs.

Where then is the meaning of sport to be found? Recall the core of the WADA Code's concise description of the "spirit of sport" (here I must confess that I had a hand in drafting this section): "the pursuit of human excellence through the dedicated perfection of each person's natural talents.... The spirit of sport is the celebration of the human spirit, body and mind, and is reflected in values we find in and through sport." There is far more to be said about the meaning of sport and the values we find there. But I believe this is a good start that reflects well why people love sport, and why they overwhelmingly prefer a sport free of doping.

Bibliography

1 Murray, T.H. The coercive power of drugs in sports. *Hastings Cent. Rep.* 1983; 13(4): 24–30. Doi:10.2307/3561718.

2 Fost, N. Banning drugs in sports: a skeptical view. *Hastings Cent. Rep.* 1986; 16(4): 5–10.

3 US Anti-Doping Agency (USADA). Cycling Investigation | US Anti-Doping Agency (USADA). http://cyclinginvestigation.usada.org/. Accessed December 16, 2013.

4 Vaughters, J. How to get doping out of sports, NYTimes.com. www.nytimes.com/2012/08/12/opinion/sunday/how-to-get-doping-out-of-sports.html. Accessed January 11, 2016.

5 McGee, B. How dopers stole the best years of my career. *Sidney Morning Herald.* October 27, 2012: 10–13.

6 Austin, S. "I quit cycling because of the drugs. Now I am Lance Armstrong's best riding buddy," www.telegraph.co.uk/sport/othersports/cycling/10562181/I-quit-cycling-because-of-the-drugs.-Now-I-am-Lance-Armstrongs-best-riding-buddy.html. Published January 9, 2014. Accessed May 5, 2015.

7 McNamee, M. Anti-anti doping: why scepticism doesn't cut the mustard. *Br. Med. J.* 2008; 337: a584.

8 Savulescu, J. Why we should allow performance enhancing drugs in sport. *Br. J. Sports Med.* 2004; 38(6): 666–670. Doi:10.1136/bjsm.2003.005249.

9 Miah, A. Enhanced athletes? It's only natural. *Wash. Post.* August 3, 2008: B1-B5.

10 FINA, *Dubai Charter.* 2009. www.fina.org/project/images/help/thedubaicharter.pdf. Accessed January 11, 2016.

11 World Anti-Doping Agency, *World Anti-Doping Code.* World Anti-Doping Agency. 2015. www.wada-ama.org/Documents/World_Anti-Doping_Program/WADP-The-Code/Code_Review/Code%20Review%202015/Code%20Final%20Draft/WADA-2015-World-Anti-Doping-Code.pdf. Accessed May 13, 2014.

12 Loland, S., Hoppeler, H. Justifying anti-doping: the fair opportunity principle and the biology of performance enhancement. *European J. Sports Science* 2012; 4: 347–353.

13 Tamburrini, C.M. What's wrong with genetic inequality? The impact of genetic technology on elite sports and society. *Sport Ethics Philos.* 2007; 1: 229–238.

14 Brown, W.M. Ethics, drugs, and sport. *J. Philos. Sport.* 1980; 7: 15–23.

15 Tännsjö, T. Hypoxic air machines: commentary. *J. Med. Ethics.* 2005; 31(2): 113–113. Doi:10.1136/jme.2003.005355.

16 Murray, T.H. In search of an ethics for sport. In: T.H. Murray, K.J. Maschke and A.A. Wasunna (eds) *Performance-Enhancing Technologies in Sports: Ethical, Conceptual, and Scientific Issues.* Baltimore: Johns Hopkins University Press; 2009: 225–238.

17 Loland, S., Murray, T.H. The ethics of the use of technologically constructed high-altitude environments to enhance performances in sport. *Scand. J. Med. Sci. Sports.* 2007; 17(3): 193–195. Doi:10.1111/j.1600–0838.2007.00653.x.

18 Murray, T.H. Doping and anti-doping: an inquiry into the meaning of sport. In: M.J. McNamee and W. Morgan (ed.) *Routledge Handbook of the Philosophy of Sport.* London: Routledge; 2015.

19 Kayser, B., Mauron, A., Miah, A. Current anti-doping policy: a critical appraisal. *BMC Med. Ethics.* 2007; 8: 1–10.

20 Kreft, L. Elite sportspersons and commodity control: anti-doping as quality assurance. *Int. J. Sport Policy Polit.* 2011; 3(2): 151–161. Doi:10.1080/19406940.2011.577795.

21 Overbye, M., Wagner, U. Experiences, attitudes and trust: an inquiry into elite athletes' perception of the whereabouts reporting system. *Int. J. Sport Policy Polit.* 2013; (May): 1–22. Doi:10.1080/19406940.2013.791712.

22 Johnson, J., Butryn, T., Masucci, M.A. A focus group analysis of the US and Canadian female triathletes' knowledge of doping. *Sport Soc.* 2013; 16(5): 654–671. Doi:10.1080/17430437.2012.753522.

23 Kayser, B., Smith, A.C.T. Globalisation of anti-doping: the reverse side of the medal. *BMJ.* 2008; 337: 85–87.

24 Hoffman, J.R., Ratamess, N.A. Medical issues associated with anabolic steroid use: are they exaggerated? *J. Sports Sci. Med.* 2006; 5: 182–193.

25 Sjoqvist, F., Garle, M., Rane, A. Use of doping agents, particularly anabolic steroids, in sports and society. *Lancet.* 2008; 371: 1872–1882.

26 US Food and Drug Administration. Public Health Advisory: erythropoiesis-stimulating agents (ESAs). www.fda.gov/ForConsumers/ByAudience/ForPatientAdvocates/HIVandAIDSActivities/ucm124262.htm. Accessed December 16, 2013.

27 Kanayama, G., Hudson, J.I. Long-term psychiatric and medical consequences of anabolic–androgenic steroid abuse: a looming public health concern? *Drug Alcohol Depend.* 2008; 98: 1–12. Doi:10.1016/j.drugalcdep. 2008.05.004.

28 Franke, W.W., Berendonk, B. Hormonal doping and androgenization of athletes: a secret program of the German Democratic Republic government. *Clin. Chem.* 1997; 43(7): 1262–1279.

29 Hoberman, J. Sports physicians and doping: medical ethics and elite performance. In: D. Malcolm and S. Parissa (eds) *The Social Organization of Sports Medicine: Critical Socio-Cultural Perspectives.* London and New York: Routledge; 2012.

30 Murray, T.H. Divided loyalties for physicians: social context and moral problems. *Soc. Sci. Med.* 1986; 23(8): 827–827.

31 Faden, R., Shebaya, S. Public health ethics. http://plato.stanford.edu/entries/publichealth-ethics/. Accessed January 11, 2016.

32 Kass, N.E. An ethics framework for public health. *Am. J. Public Health.* 2001; 91(11): 1776–1782.

33 Childress, J.F., Gaare Bernheim, R. Public health ethics: public justification and public trust. *Bundesgesundheitsblatt – Gesundheitsforschung – Gesundheitsschutz.* 2008; 51(2): 158–163. Doi:10.1007/s00103–008–0444–6.

34 Savulescu, J., Foddy, B, Clayton, M. Why we should allow performance enhancing drugs in sport. *Br. J. Sports Med.* 2004; 38.

10 The doping tug of war – from an Olympic sport to an enduring challenge to Sport and to public policy

Theodore Friedmann

Introduction and background

Doping is an ancient and familiar part of Sport. For the first two decades of the twentieth century, the tug of war was an established and formal competitive event of the early re-established modern summer Olympic games. Like most athletic events, the goal and the inevitable outcome was victory for one side or another.

Although the tug of war event itself has vanished from the Olympic Games and from elite international Sport, it has come to be replaced by an analogous but far more enduring form of tug of war: i.e., between doping and anti-doping forces in Sport. And, as recent history has suggested, this tug of war tends to conclude not in definitive victories but rather in exchanges of advances as forms of doping and cheating come to be detected and then replaced by more sophisticated and technologically updated techniques that in turn lead to anti-doping technical advances, and so on, ad infinitum.

Doping in modern Sport

Modern science has changed the face of doping. Most modern Sport – professional, amateur recreational and even scholastic – are suffused with performance-enhancing manipulations with drugs and training tools. The anti-doping community of scholars and scientists who are intent on preventing Sport from degenerating into mere engineering and biotechnological contests continue to struggle to develop powerful new methods for physicochemical detection and identification of doping agents and, increasingly, to correlate drug exposure with the complex and wide genetic and metabolic changes induced by their use. The IOC, international sports federations, the World Anti-Doping Agency (WADA), national anti-doping agencies and many professional sports organizations have begun to carry out increasingly extensive screening and monitoring programs that apply these scientific and technological advances to detect illicit use of pharmacological agents and disallowed tools and methods to ensure that doping comes to light and then to institute punitive responses in cases where doping is proven.

Concomitantly, forces intent on subverting the anti-doping movement and on applying any and all methods, legal or illegal, permitted or illicit, have continued to develop increasingly sophisticated and ever more stealthy doping agents and tools in the pursuit of allowing unfettered doping methods to provide an element of performance enhancement or at least to provide a hope of performance enhancement and thereby create a large and lucrative market demand.

Without doubt, both sides of this tug of war are continually making impressive advances. On one hand, sophisticated teams of scientists and technicians, well supported by deep covert funding sources, are continually creating new drugs completely unfamiliar to the monitoring anti-doping agencies and to the legal community. Such teams often merely chemically modify existing agents to make them undetectable by established testing methods and, in the course of that work, not only provide performance enhancement and lucrative careers for athletes, their retinues and sponsors but concomitantly put the careers of non-doping athletes at a severe disadvantage and, in many cases, destroy the careers of honest and non-doping athletes. This side of the contest has even been joined by the pro-doping sport philosophy community (1–3) that maintains that it is permissible, even ethically required, to permit the use of any and all drug-based and even surgical reconstruction methods and tools (including nonsensical support for constructing webbing between the fingers and toes of swimmers to increase stroke power) while giving only reluctant and glancing recognition of the damage that such an approach does, not only to the valued and deeply human role that Sport plays in all human societies but also to the great potential harm to the health of athletes, whether they be elite international stars, recreational athletes or even children aspiring to become serious athletes.

On the other hand, the anti-doping and monitoring communities are taking advantage of remarkable improvements in the tools and methods used for detection of doping agents and, in particular, in the use of new genetic and genomic tools to identify the genetic signatures that are the inevitable results of exposure to performance-enhancing agents (4, 5). Advances on one side are counterbalanced by increasing resistance and often equally impressive advances, illicit as they might be, on the other side.

A long-term outlook for the doping tug of war

Our changing view of Sport makes a purely technological solution to doping unlikely. One would hope that there could be a solution to the seductive social forces that lure athletes and nations into doping with reward and even illegal drug- or genetically enhanced doping and cheating in Sport. Sadly, that possibility seems unlikely. In the absence of an improbable massive changes to our social concept of Sport as glorious honest athletic competition but rather increasingly as entertainment, major international business, commerce and even as a belligerent national competition for prestige, an end to this tug of war between doping and anti-doping will remain elusive.

Major new directions in the development of illicit doping agents and tools

Continuing advances in technology make the tools of doping ever more efficient. The revelation during the past several decades of widespread major doping activities in Sport has provided powerful proof for the existence of a thriving and aggressive cottage industry intent on making molecular modifications to existing doping agents and on producing novel agents for which no chemical or biological detection tools yet exist. This doping industry has moved far beyond its early history of using relatively simple chemical and easily detectable agents to a phase now characterized by the application of highly sophisticated concepts of drug design by expert and highly trained molecular biologists, synthetic chemists and physiologists familiar with current detection methods and capable of designing and producing derivatives and new agents that are undetectable by current tools. The success of these doping efforts and consortia is attested to by recent history of very high visibility world-class athletes who are subjected repeatedly to monitoring and detection programs but who nevertheless succeed for years and even decades to avoid detection through the development of pharmacologically and physiologically clever administration strategies and by using newly and custom-developed agents. Industries devoted to improving chemical and biological detection instruments and methods are at a disadvantage compared to those whose single aim is to identify weaknesses and deficiencies in instrumentation technology or to make chemical modifications that allow doping agents to become invisible to detection tools while retaining their biological action. It seems inevitable that direct chemical detection of any doping agent will meet with such countermeasures by determined chemists and biologists. As chemical methods of detection improve, so will chemical methods to mask their detectability.

Major new directions in the development of more powerful methods to combat and detect doping in Sport

Just as in the case of new doping tools, evolving technology makes doping detection increasingly effective. Advances in molecular genetics over the past several decades have pointed to two areas in which modern molecular genetic approaches will greatly alter the landscape of doping itself. In the first place, genetics has the potential to enable attempts to carry out doping through the expression in athletes of foreign genes that express functions able to enhance athletic performance ("gene doping") by providing powerful new routes toward doping itself. In addition, the tools of molecular genetics have the potential to vastly improve the ability to detect doping whether it be the result of drug- or gene-based doping.

In addition to improvements in chemical and instrumentation methods for detecting doping (6), there has been a major new approach based on finding changes in gene expression that accompany the exposure to doping agents and methods – the so-called search for genetic "signatures" of doping.

Gene-based doping

The use of genes and genetic elements is a potentially powerful new approach to doping. The potential use of powerful modern tools for genetic manipulation for the purposes of treating disease suggest strongly that it will become feasible in the near future to introduce foreign genes into tissues of athletes to enhance physiological functions with sufficient efficiency to permit enhancement of physical performance. This conclusion comes directly from recent major advances in the use of gene transfer methods to correct certain kinds of human genetic disease; i.e., gene therapy. In some cases, disorders such as primary immunodeficiency, a growing number of genetic forms of blindness, hemophilia, forms of cancer and other genetic disorders have been corrected, possibly even "cured," thereby permitting a great improvement in quality of life for patients with otherwise intractable diseases. The concept of gene therapy lies in the conceptually simple but technically difficult task of replacing or restoring the function of a gene responsible for a human disease. In principle, correction of such gene defects at the appropriate time during development can prevent or even reverse the progress of a genetic disease. It is very likely that the same concept can and will be applied not to correct a genetic defect but rather to add a new genetic function to tissues that play a vital role in an athletic function and thereby to enhance the function of such tissues and provide an advantage to athletic performance. It was the fore-sightedness of Prof. Arne Ljungqvist at the IOC and then at the newly organized WADA who first recognized the need for a peremptory regulatory response to this impending problem and who established the area of gene doping as an area of special emphasis for the research program of the Health, Medicine and Research Committee early in the development of WADA.

During the past several years, even more remarkable advances have been made in the search for methods to modify existing genes or to introduce new genetic functions into the human genome, both in vitro and even in vivo. One of the requirements for genetic modifications in humans is the need to carry out such changes with perfect specificity and precision so as not to interfere with the other tens of thousands of human genes to disturb normal functions. Recently, several such methods have been developed and have introduced entirely new urgency to define and solve the scientific dilemmas of human genetic modification, not only for possible disease treatment and prevention and enhancement of normal functions such as those that determine athletic capability, but also to prepare for the inevitable and more ominous uses with eugenic potential.

These powerful new methods constitute the new field of genome "editing" (7–10) and go by the names of Zinc-finger, TALEN and CRISPR/Cas9 technology. They permit the modification of endogenous DNA sequence from abnormal to normal sequences and the addition of new genes into very specific sites in the genome to minimize and potentially eliminate the potential for unwanted changes in normal and essential genes. For the first time, it is now potentially possible to design and carry out specific genetic changes in the human that leave no "foot-print" and no clues for genetic changes having been made. The current pressures for developing these methods are obviously those related to the prevention and treatment of disease, but as in the case of all genetic modification technology, they will be applied to enhancement attempts to alter normal functions and thereby improve quality of life. Of course, the technology is very early and experimental and will require very extensive improvements of efficiency and safety before they can be ready for application for human genetic modification. But the disease-related applications are developing with great speed and temptations will develop to extend uses to broader normal human functions such as athletic and other quality of life long before we are ready, technically, ethically or societally.

Although many genes can become candidates for gene doping, the genes most commonly envisioned for this kind of gene-based doping are (1) genes that regulate muscle growth and function such as human growth hormone, insulin-like growth factors (IGF-1), myostatin and other growth factors associated with muscle growth and function, and (2) genes such as erythropoietin that regulate erythrocyte production and thereby control the efficiency of oxygen delivery and toxic metabolites in exercising organs and tissues. It is relatively easy to imagine how such genes can be used in the world of Sport because expression of these classes of genes has been successful in animal models including rodents and non-human primates, producing marked increase in muscle growth and function in the case of IGF-1 and great increase in erythrocyte production and oxygen-carrying capacity in the case of erythropoietin. These kinds of agents are, of course, well known to doping athletes and anti-doping agencies because they are already in common use in their form as gene products – protein hormones and growth factors. While application to humans would seem to be straightforward, there are many important caveats dealing with safety – such manipulations in test animals can and have been shown to have disastrous and even life-threatening consequences. Even in the case of authentic gene therapy studies, the manipulations are subject to very heavy levels of governmental oversight and regulation because of their highly experimental nature and the risk for potentially dangerous unintended consequences. Sadly, those who are likely to underwrite and push for genetic manipulations in Sport are unlikely to be concerned about complying with the universal ethical precepts such those represented by the Helsinki Declarations of the World Medical Association and many other national and international standards for the protection of human subjects that underlie acceptable and ethical experimentation with human subjects.

Despite persistent rumors and suspicions, there is no incontrovertible evidence yet that these or any other gene-based modifications have been carried out or even attempted in Sport. However, the temptations for illicit use of these methods in Sport are very great and the high likelihood that they will indeed be used relatively soon is underscored by the aborted attempt in 2006 by the German athletic trainer Thomas Springstein to obtain a gene-transfer agent that had been developed to introduce a functioning EPO gene into patients with cancer and chronic kidney disease (11). It's not likely that Mr Springstein was planning to carry out a clinical study with such patients. The technology of expressing foreign genes in human beings not only for therapeutic purposes but also for life-style and sport applications is racing ahead and the rewards for successful application to functions relevant to sport performance are far too alluring to ignore.

Detection of gene-based doping

The tools potentially useful for gene-based doping may be turned around and used to detect the existence and expression of a foreign, performance-enhancing gene. Methods for the detection of doping agents based on physical identification of such agents in accessible body fluids from athletes suffer from the problems associated with the ever-more sophisticated tools available to the doping community to hide such agents with molecular modification of the agents masking agents, with design and synthesis of novel compounds not yet susceptible to chemical detection, and with physiologically sophisticated dosages and dosage schedules. During the past decade, largely through the impetus provided by the WADA research program, a new approach to doping detection has arisen that in principle should be much less vulnerable to the kinds of molecular modification or biosynthetic techniques mentioned above. The concept underlying this approach is based on the identification of the many inevitable homeostatic biochemical or genetic changes in tissue or biological fluids that result from exposure to a doping agent, whether it be a pharmacological or genetic agent. Agents such as growth hormones, erythropoietin and probably all other doping agents or tools would be expected to produce very broad effects on many systems of physiological function and patterns of gene expression as they produce the desired effect in a doping setting and as the body's homeostatic mechanisms work to counteract the perturbations of the doping agent. A pattern of those changes central to the desired physiological effect should be readily detectable as system-wide changes in the expression of a large number of genetic and biochemical functions and should therefore constitute a "signature" of previous exposure to a genetic or pharmacological agent. No matter how well the original doping agent may be disguised or made undetectable by available physical detection tools, it is safe to assume that many of the broad systems effects will have been expressed if the desired effects of the agent are to be achieved. It seems very unlikely that such a large number of diverse components of the altered genetic signature will be easily subject to masking in reversal.

The identification of genetic signatures of doping has been spearheaded by WADA with special emphasis on human growth hormone and erythropoietin. Recent studies with these agents both in animal model studies and in human subjects have given highly encouraging support for this approach to the detection of exposure to doping agents and have brought the anti-doping world close to rigorous in-field tests of such an approach. An area in which progress has been particularly impressive is in the demonstration of a strong genetic signature for doping with erythropoietin (Epo). The studies of Yannis Pitsiladis (12–13) have shown that exposure of world-class as well as recreational athletes to Epo results in dysregulated expression of multiple genes that, in the aggregate, constitute a strong presumptive signature for Epo. Another advance has come from the detection of some virus vectors used to introduce performance-altering genes into athletes (14, 15). These new tools in the anti-doping armamentarium help to even the playing field between the doping and anti-doping teams in the tug of war but we all realize that advances and improvements will take place on both sides of the rope. The tug of war match is not over.

The need for more research

The world of Sport, from elite to amateur, needs a consistent, stable and well-supported mechanism for the pursuit of research to counter the growing sophistication of the doping community. The terrain of doping and anti-doping is changing drastically and quickly. Although impressive progress has been made in the development of new concepts and tools for the effort to detect and deter doping, the task remains to anticipate and then respond to the new and unfortunately effective doping methods being constantly developed. The time is approaching rapidly when the powerful new tools of genetic signatures of exposure to doping agents will be at hand and will pose immense new kinds of problems that those intent on obfuscating anti-doping technology will find it very difficult to accomplish. But the need for powerful and more effective new concepts and tools for the battle against doping in Sport will require a greater and more stable level of funding for anti-doping research, as was recently emphasized by the new IOC president Thomas Bach in preparation for the Olympic Games in Sochi, Russia. He has challenged nations to be prepared to match an increase in IOC funding to the research program at WADA so that innovative anti-doping techniques can be developed and implemented quickly. That kind of research will be difficult, time-consuming and expensive. But it is a necessary investment in the effort to preserve clean and honest Sport and to augment the effectiveness of the public health protections not only for athletes but for the entire society. It is encouraging that the IOC and WADA (14, 15) have announced increased funding for the anti-doping effort – a great catalyst to the anti-doping effort.

Doping is a symptom of a larger public health threat

Doping is not only a problem for Sport, but also a major public health problem. Doping is increasingly coming to be recognized not only as a problem for Sport but rather as a symptom of a much broader society-wide threat to many other human activities and to human health (16). The most obvious threat to public health posed by doping lies in the increasing use of doping agents and tools by growing children who have aspirations to become athletes. Many of the well-known doping agents are known to have deleterious effects on many developing physiological systems and the urge to emulate sport heroes will certainly put these young lives in jeopardy. Of course, drugs are playing a legitimate and vital role in medicine, in saving lives and in improving the quality of life for most humans. However, the pervasive use of drugs for non-therapeutic purposes carries with it the danger of replacing human effort and creativity with biotechnological phenomenology. Sport is one of the most important testing grounds for these kinds of effects and represents a canary in the coal mine of human society. Being alert to the existence and consequences of doping in Sport provides scientific and social avenues to allow our society to learn how to take advantage of pharmacological science for the public good while anticipating and averting the harms of replacing basic human functions with drugs.

References

1 Kayser, B., Mauron, A. and Miah, A. Current anti-doping policy: a critical appraisal. *BMC Med. Ethics* 2007 (March 29); 8: 2.
2 Fost, N. "Doping" is pejorative and misleading. *BMJ* 2008 (July 22); 337: a910; doi: 10.1136/bmj.a910.
3 Tierney, J. What's natural about Olympic athletes? *New York Times* (August 13, 2008).
4 Friedmann, T., Rabin, O. and Frankel, M.S. Ethics. Gene doping and sport. *Science* 2010 (February 5); 327(5966): 647–648. Doi: 10.1126/science.1177801.
5 Friedmann, T. How close are we to gene doping? *Hastings Cent. Rep.* 2010 (March–April); 40(2): 20–22.
6 Friedmann, T., Flenker, U., Georgakopoulos, C., Alsayrafi, M., Sottas, P.E., Williams, S.A. and Gill, R.D. Evolving concepts and techniques for anti-doping. *Bioanalysis* 2012 (July); 4(13): 1667–1680. Doi: 10.4155/bio.12.146.
7 Heckl, D. and Charpentier, E. Toward whole-transcriptome editing with CRISPR-Cas9. *Mol. Cell.* 2015 (May 21); 58(4): 560–562. Doi: 10.1016/j.molcel.2015.05.016.
8 Dance, A. Core concept: CRISPR gene editing. *Proc. Natl Acad. Sci. USA* 2015 (May 19); 112(20): 6245–6246. Doi: 10.1073/pnas.1503840112.
9 Hossain, M.A., Barrow, J.J., Shen, Y., Haq, M.I. and Bungert, J. Artificial zinc finger DNA binding domains: versatile tools for genome engineering and modulation of gene expression. *J. Cell. Biochem.* 2015 (May 18). Doi: 10.1002/jcb.25226.
10 Biffi, A. Clinical translation of TALENS: treating SCID-X1 by gene editing in iPSCs. *Cell Stem Cell* 2015 (April 2); 16(4): 348–349. Doi: 10.1016/j.stem.2015.03.009.
11 Schofield, M. East Germany's doping legacy lives on, 25 years later. McClatchy Foreign Staff (February 13, 2015).
12 Pitsiladis, Y.P., Durussel, J. and Rabin, O. An integrative "omics" solution to the detection of recombinant human erythropoietin and blood doping. *Br. J. Sports Med.* 2014 (May); 48 (10): 856–861. Doi: 10.1136/bjsports-2014–093529 (review).
13 Dvorak, J., Saugy, M. and Pitsiladis, Y.P. Challenges and threats to implementing the fight against doping in sport. *Br. J. Sports Med.* 2014 (May); 48 (10): 807–809; doi: 10.1136/bjsports-2014–093589.
14 www.wada-ama.org/en/media/news/2015-04/pcc-and-wada-form-anti-doping-research-partnership.
15 www.olympic.org/news/call-for-applications-anti-doping-research-fund/235010.
16 www.arneljungqvist.com/the-foundation/patron.

Index

Page numbers in *italics* denote tables, those in **bold** denote figures.